Color Atlas of
Plastering Techniques

Color Atlas of
Plastering Techniques

Kenneth Mills
MA, BSc, FRCS
Consultant Orthopaedic Surgeon
Grampian Health Board, Aberdeen
Scotland

Graham Page
ChM, FRCS, MB, ChB,
Consultant in Accident and Emergency Care
Grampian Health Board, Aberdeen
Scotland

Richard Morton
MSc, FRPS, FBPA, AIMBI
Director, Graves Medical Audiovisual Library
Chelmsford, Essex
England

MEDICAL ECONOMICS BOOKS
Oradell, New Jersey 07649

Copyright © K. Mills, G. Page, R. Morton 1986
Published by Wolfe Medical Publications Ltd 1986
Printed by W.S. Cowell Ltd, 8 Buttermarket, Ipswich,
England.

Distributed in North America by Medical Economics
Company, Oradell, New Jersey, by arrangement with
Wolfe Medical Publications Ltd

Library of Congress Cataloging in Publication Data

Mills, K. L. G. (Kenneth L. G.)
    Color atlas of plastering techniques.

    Spine title: Plastering techniques.
    1. Plaster casts, Surgical—Atlases.   2. Plastering—
Technique—Atlases.   I. Page, Graham.   II. Morton,
Richard.   III. Title.   [DNLM: 1. Casts, Surgical—
atlases.   2. Plastering techniques.   WO   517   M657c]
RD114.M55   1986   617′.15   85-13897
ISBN 0-87489-423-9

Acknowledgements

Our thanks are due to the following plaster technicians without whom this book could not have been compiled – Denis Buyers, Albert Hendry, Elizabeth Pickard, Doreen Abel and our models, also to Sister A M Gibbs and the Staff of the Accident and Emergency Department, Royal Infirmary, Aberdeen.

Introduction

Plaster of Paris bandage and its modern equivalents are applied to patients all over the world whenever there is a need to immobilise the skeleton. This book illustrates the techniques of application and aims to help plaster technicians, nurses and medical staff.

The techniques illustrated are not the only methods of achieving the desired objectives; most centres will have their preferred variations. This book shows some techniques currently in use in Aberdeen. Not every type of plaster has been shown; the construction of plaster beds has been omitted.

Plaster of Paris

Plaster of Paris takes its name from Paris, France, where it was first widely used chemically, surgically and constructionally. However, one of the earliest surgical uses was recorded in 1852 when A. Mathyson, a Dutch Army Surgeon, rubbed powdered plaster into cotton bandages to form splints.

Plaster of Paris, in its raw state, is termed gypsum – hydrated calcium sulphate with impurities. The surgical form is pure anhydrous calcium sulphate. The essential chemical step is the heating of gypsum to 120°C (250°F).

$$2(Ca\,SO_4 \cdot 2H_2O) \gtrless (Ca\,SO_4)_2 \cdot H_2O + 3H_2O$$

Adding water allows for a return to the original crystalline state of full hydration. Twenty per cent of added water is incorporated into the hydrated crystal lattice but the other 80% of water eventually evaporates. The absorption of water while setting gives out heat (an exothermic reaction) but not enough to cause discomfort or injury.

Advantages
Plaster of Paris is extremely safe and does not produce allergies. It is infinitely adaptable to the part being splinted and can be applied speedily without gloves. It is cheap in comparison with more modern materials.

Disadvantages
Plaster of Paris is slow to dry, to gain full strength and is seriously weakened if it becomes wet again. It is very heavy when wet but becomes much lighter when dry. It is partially radio-opaque, obscuring bone detail on radiographs.

Mechanical characteristics
Low temperatures and sugar solutions retard setting while high temperatures and salt or borax solutions accelerate it. The setting time is three times longer at 5°C (40°F) than at 50°C (125°F). Although setting takes only a few minutes, drying may take many hours – roughly 36 hours for an arm cast, 48-60 hours for a leg cast and up to 7 days for a hip spica, especially if the atmosphere is moist and cool. Movement of the plaster while it is setting will cause gross weakening. The optimum strength is achieved when it is completely dry (but as mentioned there is still a water content of 20% within the crystalline structure). Mechanical failure of a cast is due to the different elastic moduli in gauze fibres and hydrated calcium sulphate.

Alternatives to plaster of Paris

The past 15 years have seen a rapid development of various fibreglass and resinous materials which can be safely applied as external splints. These are light, durable and waterproof but require protective packaging and are difficult to apply without wearing gloves. They do not splash like plaster of Paris but may require the application of a wet cotton bandage on the exterior to improve conformity while hardening occurs over periods of 10-30 minutes. They are hardened by exposure to water and/or light. They are considerably more expensive than plaster at present, but to balance this disadvantage, fewer bandages are required and they are much more durable and so are particularly suitable for active or elderly patients. They are more radiolucent than plaster.

A number of preformed plastic components are available as an alternative to plaster. They are made to fit different sizes of limbs and to allow movement at joints. They remain experimental and are not considered further in this book.

Contents

TECHNIQUES

Application of a plaster cast

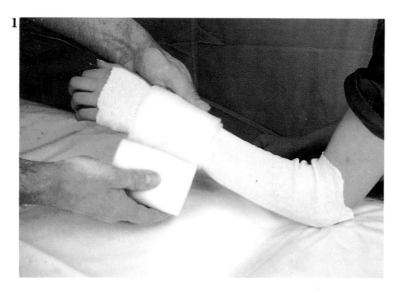

1 The injured limb is prepared for application of plaster by covering the skin with tubular gauze to protect the hairs and a layer of padding to allow for swelling and to protect the bony prominences.

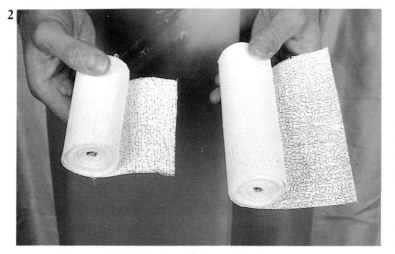

2 Rolls of plaster bandage 10 and 15 cm (4 and 6 in) wide and 3 m (3 yards) long.

3 The plaster bandage is unwound for 10 cm (4 in) and both the roll and the free end are held under the water for a few seconds until bubbles cease to rise. Cold water is used to extend the setting time and hot water to shorten it.

4 The plaster bandage is lifted out of the water and gently squeezed or the bandage drawn between finger and thumb to wring out the water. It can then be wrapped around the part to be splinted.

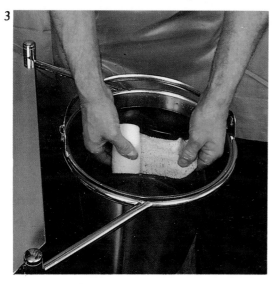

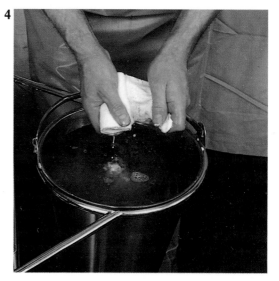

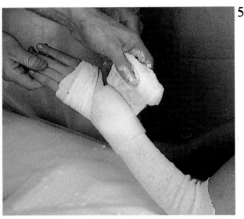

5 The wet plaster bandage is *applied distally* and *proceeds proximally*; this diminishes venous congestion and allows smoother application of the bandage. An overlap of padding 1-2 cm (½-¾ in) wide should be left to protrude beyond the margins of the plaster.

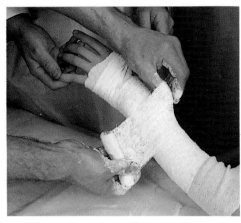

6 Where a limb circumference enlarges, the circles of wet plaster bandage are gussetted or tucked in as shown. A 50% overlap of width gives a double layer of plaster, a 60% overlap gives a triple layer.

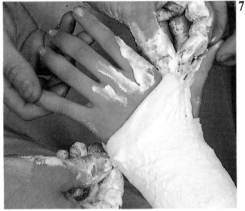

7 At the distal free edge the gauze and padding are turned back to give a smooth edge. The knuckle joints are allowed full movement.

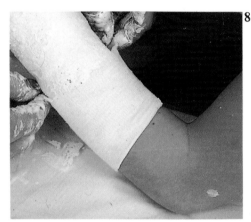

8 At the proximal free edge the gauze and padding are also turned back. The plaster edge is adjusted to allow free flexion of the elbow.

9 The plaster cast is smoothed and moulded to fit the limb accurately. The injured limb should be elevated in a high sling or on pillows at the bedside. The circulation is checked regularly. If the patient goes home shortly after application he is asked to return the next day for inspection of the limb and the cast. Most units give their patients a printed list of danger signals and instructions about seeking advice. Information about care of the cast and exercises for the limb is usually included.

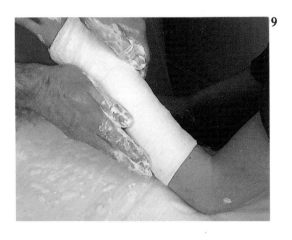

Application of a plaster splint (slab)

Plaster splints (slabs) are used for the following. (1) *Initial splinting* of fractures and other injuries. They are easily applied and allow more space for swelling of the limb than a circular plaster cast. (2) *Reinforcement* of circular plaster casts to strengthen weak points, e.g. at a joint.

Multiple layers of plaster bandage are available in commercial preparations for preparing splints. The required length can be pulled out of the box and cut off.

Alternatively a roll of plaster is unrolled on a flat dry surface and doubled backwards and forwards on itself to form a splint of the required length and thickness.

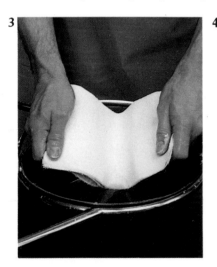

1 The limb is measured so that the correct length of splint can be prepared.

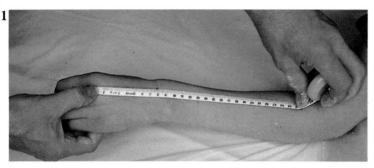

2 The required length of plaster splint is pulled out from its container.

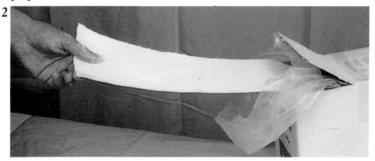

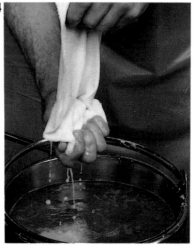

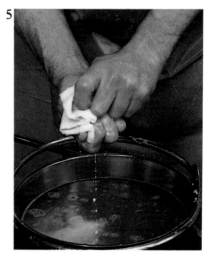

3 The splint is held at both ends and dipped in the water until the bubbles cease to rise.

4 The plaster splint is held vertically at both ends to drain off surplus water.

5 The remaining excess water is gently squeezed out of the splint by dropping the upper hand on to the lower.

7-9 The injured limb has been prepared by applying tubular gauze and padding to protect the skin and skeletal prominences. The wet plaster splint is laid on the padding leaving the distal and proximal 1- 2 cm (½-¾ in) free of padding (**7**). These are turned back later to form a smooth edge. The splint is held in place by a wet cotton bandage which is applied with even tension, working distally to proximally (**8**). (This direction helps to diminish swelling of the hand or foot.) The plaster splint is completed with proximal and distal edges turned back and smoothly held in place by the exterior bandage. The knuckles are allowed complete freedom and the elbow can be fully flexed without the proximal edge digging into the flesh (**9**). In the leg the toes are left free and the top edge of the plaster cast must allow for full knee flexion.

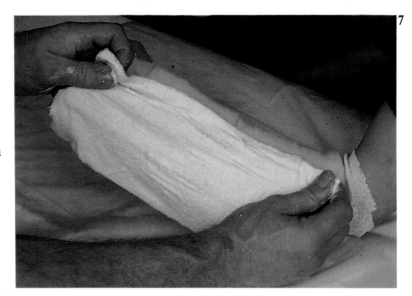

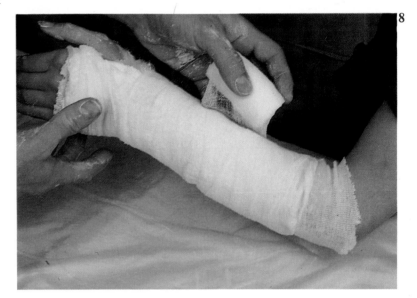

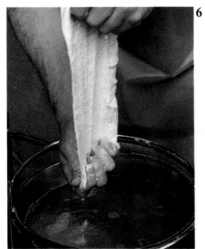

6 The hands are separated drawing out the wet splint to its full length.

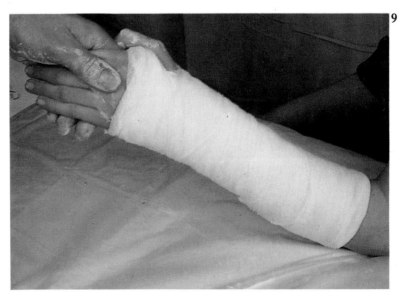

Removal of a plaster cast and splint (slab)

A plaster splint (slab) can be removed easily by using a pair of scissors to cut the gauze padding and bandage on the side of the limb opposite to the plaster. Complete circular plasters are more difficult to remove as there is a possibility of damaging the patient's skin. It is an advantage to have an assistant to hold the plaster steady in case of inadvertent movement by the patient.

The oscillating saw, of which there are several models, is widely used for removal of plaster casts.

Patients, particularly children, are afraid of being cut by the saw and dislike the noise. Efforts should be made to gain their confidence. It does not damage skin, provided it is not tethered by plaster holding the hairs etc., or unless the skin is very thin and fragile, as in patients with rheumatoid arthritis. Serious damage can be caused to an unconscious patient and great care must be exercised in this circumstance.

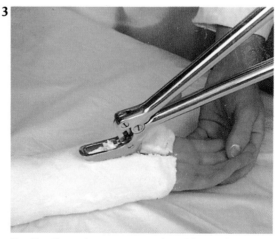

1   Tools for removal of a plaster cast. A, Benders; B, Small shears; C, Large shears; D, Plaster scissors; E, Oscillating saw. There are a number of other tools in use in plaster rooms which are not illustrated here.

16

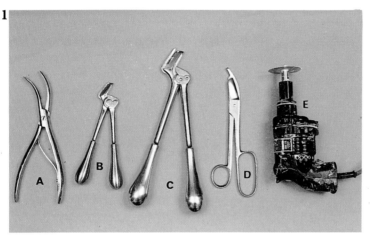

2   Removal of a plaster cast by shears requires the help of an assistant to hold the limb steady. A line of cut is chosen which will avoid any skeletal prominences. The blade is carefully introduced between the plaster and skin.

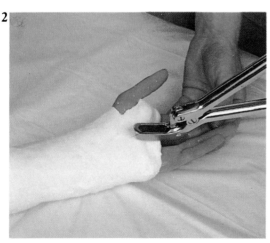

3   Small regular cuts are made, without digging the point or the heel of the blade into the patient's skin.

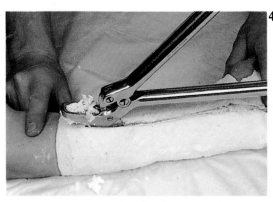

4 The assistant stretches the skin to avoid damage from the point of the shears when approaching the soft flesh of the exit point.

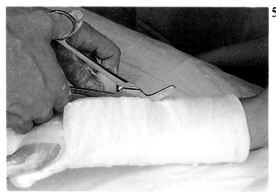

5 A plaster splint is removed by cutting through the bandages, padding and gauze with scissors on the side of the limb opposite the plaster. The same technique can be used to decompress a limb if swelling occurs.

6-9 The oscillating saw should be held so that there is no danger of the blade coming into contact with the skin (**6**). Only the plaster is cut; gauze and padding will oscillate with the blade and will not be divided. The blade quickly becomes hot in dry plaster and should be gradually rotated to use a cooler part. This short leg cast shows the lines of cutting to allow bivalving (**7**). When using the saw the blade must always be moved away from the cable to avoid damaging it. The two halves of cast can be separated by using the spreaders (**8**). On removing part of a bivalved cast, care must be taken not to angulate a mobile fracture site or a stiff joint. The back half of a cast is useful for transferring the patient for radiography (for radiographs out of plaster) and for providing a removable splint to allow intermittent joint movement.

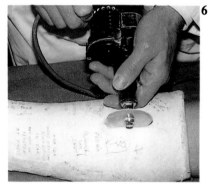

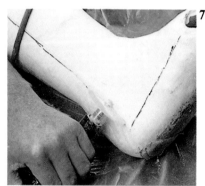

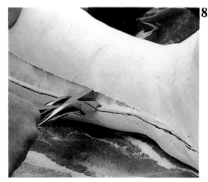

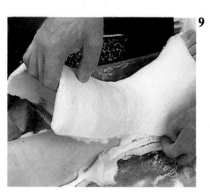

17

10 A plaster cast prevents the normal desquamation of skin and very scaly epidermis is revealed when a cast is removed after a few weeks. This can be softened by a skin emollient and soon flakes off after several washes.

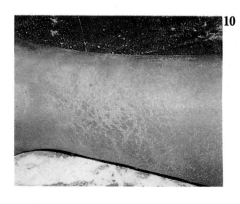

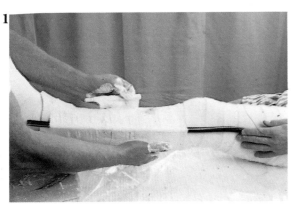

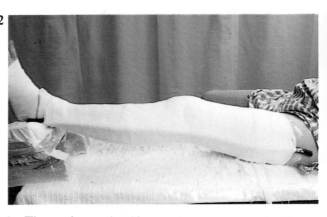

1 This technique eases the subsequent removal of a cast. A length of well greased rubber tubing is laid along the limb outside the gauze and padding.

2 The cast is completed in a routine manner covering the rubber tubing but allowing one end to protrude by 15-30 cm (6-12 in).

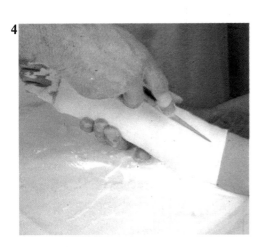

3 The tubing can be pulled out after the plaster has set. This leaves a long empty hollow in the cast, allowing easy entry for the blade of the shears when removal is required.

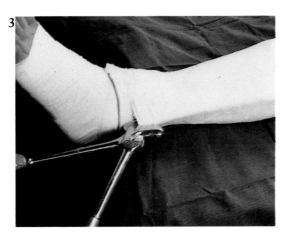

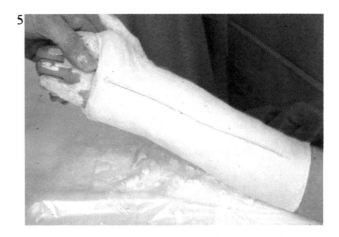

4 & 5 If a complete plaster cast is being applied to give maximum support to a recent injury or operation site there is danger of subsequent swelling causing ischaemic pain. This can be overcome by cutting the wet plaster with a sharp knife (**4**) immediately after application and if necessary separating the edges. Great care is required to avoid cutting the skin. The cut through the wet plaster can stop short of the distal and proximal edges of the cast (**5**). If swelling or pain require the cast to be split, the remaining edges can be easily divided by shears and the padding beneath the plaster cut by a pair of scissors. Skin should be seen throughout the length of the cast so that no remaining strands of padding, gauze or swabs can exert a tourniquet effect.

Windowing a plaster cast

This procedure is used to cut out parts of a cast to relieve local pressure over soft tissues or to allow access to a wound. The first step is to outline the size of the window. This should be planned from knowledge of the wound before it was encased in plaster and from radiographic evidence of the position and state of the fracture site. The window should be made a little larger than the underlying wound or pressure point. If the window is too small other rectangles of plaster must be cut out to expose the wound and these are difficult to replace satisfactorily. The rectangle of plaster should be retained and later replaced over a layer of padding and held in place with several circular turns of plaster bandage. If this is not done a rectangle of oedematous skin may result causing subsequent delay in healing. Replacement also helps to strengthen the partly opened plaster cast. If the window of plaster is unduly soiled or soft, a new one can be made from a small slab of plaster cut to size.

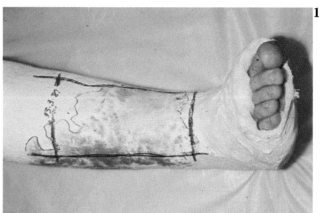

1 The outline of the window is marked on the cast.

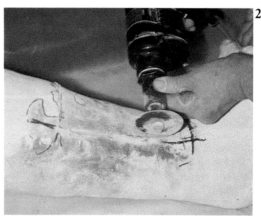

2 The blade of the saw should be supported so that it will not come in contact with the skin. The blade should be rotated gradually thus allowing the hot part of the blade to cool.

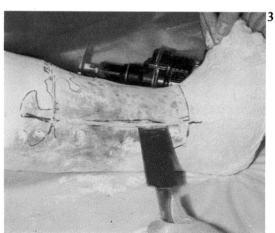

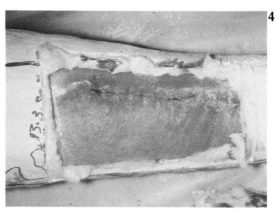

3 The rectangular plaster window is levered out of place.

4 This window is a little too small and slightly misplaced in relation to the underlying wound. Some enlargement distally and medially is required to allow removal of the stitches and application of a new dressing. The window is replaced at the end of the procedure and held in place by circular turns of plaster bandage [10 or 15 cm (4 or 6 in)].

Wedging a plaster cast

This procedure is used to correct minor degrees of malalignment of a fracture or operation site. It can be performed with minimal discomfort to the patient provided it is carried out slowly and steadily. Angles up to 30° can be corrected in this way. The plaster cast should be perfectly dry and hard otherwise the wedges will sink into the cut surfaces of wet plaster. The procedure is best performed close to an X-ray unit so that the correct position of the proposed cut can be defined and the final position after insertion of wooden wedges can be confirmed. Opening wedges are much easier to manage than closing wedges.

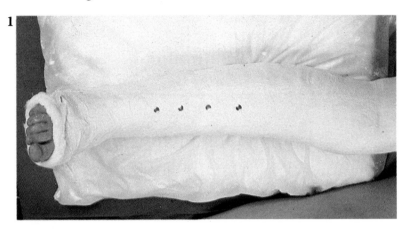

1   Radiopaque markers are placed near the site of the projected cut in the plaster. Drawing pins (thumb tacks) or paper clips are suitable. A radiograph will now allow the cut to be sited accurately.

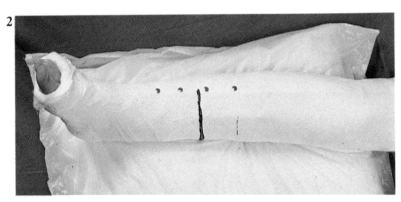

2   An ink mark is made on the plaster cast to outline the intended cut.

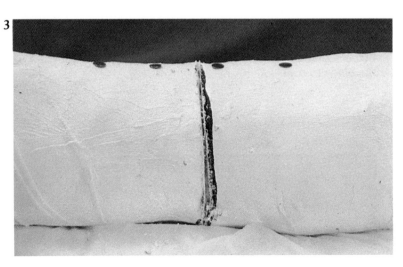

3   The plaster cast is cut down to the underlying padding or gauze over the ink mark. Two thirds of the circumference of the cast must be cut.

4 The plaster cast is gently and steadily manipulated to gradually open the cut. This should not hurt the patient.

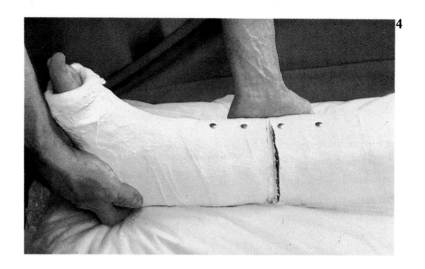

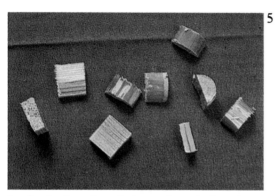

5 A selection of small pieces of wood of varying shapes and sizes [0.5-2 cm (¼-¾ in)] should be available.

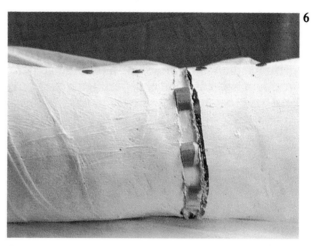

6 The wood fragments are inserted at the required degree of opening and new radiographs are taken to confirm satisfactory realignment of the fracture.

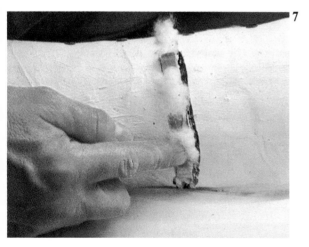

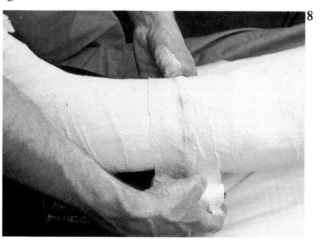

7 If the new position of the fractured bones is correct, the gaps between the wooden edges are packed with padding; this will prevent patches of oedema developing in the underlying skin.

8 The plaster cast is reinforced by a roll of plaster bandage wrapped around the site of the wedging.

APPLICATIONS

Ankle strapping

Splintage of the ankle and foot for soft tissue injuries and healing fractures can be achieved by applying elastic adhesive tape of various types. If the patient is allergic to adhesives, then elastic tubular gauze or an elastic or crepe bandage can be substituted.

Requirements Tubular gauze stocking; 1 roll elastic adhesive tape 7.5 cm × 3 m (3 in × 3 yards).

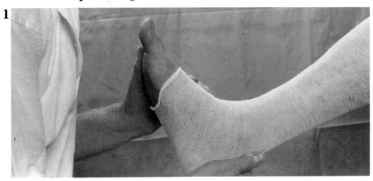

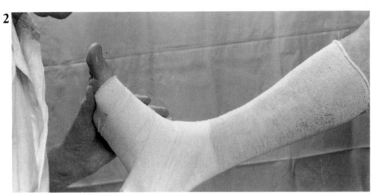

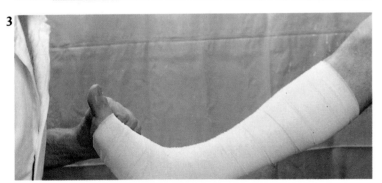

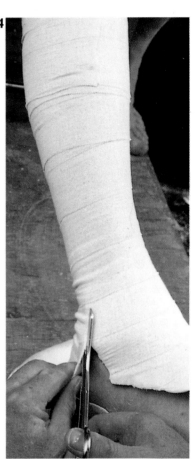

1-3 The tubular gauze stocking is fitted to the leg to protect most of the hairs and the skin from the adhesive tape. However, the stocking falls well short of the toes and the knee so that the adhesive tape can take purchase at the top and bottom margins. The patient most conveniently sits on a table or high chair so that the lower leg is suspended. The applicator sits facing the patient on a low chair or stool. The adhesive elastic tape should be applied to the skin and gauze, starting distally and moving proximally. Stretching should be avoided since it may result in ischaemia and pain. Overlapping 50% of the width at each turn gives a double layer of tape. It should be applied carefully to lie smoothly around the heel. The completed support allows freedom for the toes, a plantigrade position for the foot, and complete freedom for knee bending.

4 Removal of adhesive strapping is facilitated by the use of the gauze stocking, only a band of adhesive at the top and bottom has to be separated from the underlying skin. A strong pair of scissors with a horizontal tip to the lower blade is inserted along the lateral aspect of the foot and up the leg behind the lateral malleolus.

Knee compression bandage

Compression bandaging of the knee is frequently applied after an injury or operation to minimise swelling and to give some support and splintage. It was popularised by Robert Jones in the first decade of the 20th Century. Generally patients wearing this type of bandage should lie for long periods with their leg elevated to prevent swelling of the lower leg and to prevent the bandage sliding down the leg. Short periods of standing or walking with crutches, however, are not usually harmful. Some patients who have a knee compression bandage applied in the presence of swelling of the lower leg will need an elastic tubular stocking over the foot and leg to prevent any further swelling distal to the compression bandage. Care must be taken if rubberised elastic bandages are applied as they can produce marked compression of the knee with pain and peripheral swelling of the lower leg if they are applied too tightly.

Requirements 1 large roll of cotton wool padding; 2 or 3 15 cm (6 in) crepe bandages.

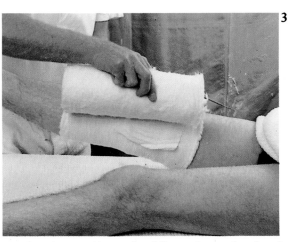
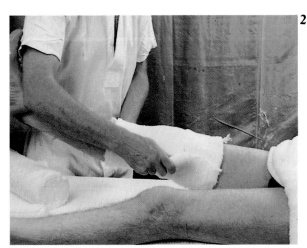

1 & 2 The foot is elevated by an assistant and the knee extended. A layer of padding is laid around extending 20 cm (8 in) above and below the knee. A 15 cm (6 in) crepe bandage is wrapped firmly over the layer of padding starting distally and ending proximally. Other types of non-elastic bandage can be used with equally good effect.

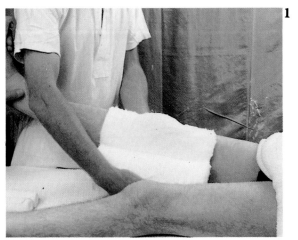
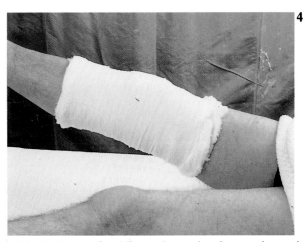

3 & 4 A second layer of padding and crepe bandage is applied (a third layer of padding and crepe bandage can be used if the padding is thin). Too bulky a compression bandage may prevent a patient wearing trousers without splitting the leg seam. The outer layer of crepe bandage can be re-applied if it loosens. Some surgeons advocate daily removal and re-application of this outer layer.

Short leg cast: plaster

This type of cast is applied to support operations or fractures about the ankle and foot. If it is necessary to eliminate rotary stresses around the ankle, the short leg cast should be extended into a Sarmiento or long leg cast. If general anaesthesia is necessary the patient lies supine with the leg supported by 2 assistants – one holding the thigh, the other the toes.

Alternatively the lower leg can be bent at the knee and hung vertically over the end or side of the table.

Requirements   1 leg stocking of tubular gauze; 1 roll of 10 cm (4 in) padding bandage; 6 rolls of 10 cm (4 in) plaster bandage; 1 splint of 10 cm (4 in) plaster bandage 10 layers thick, 20 cm long.

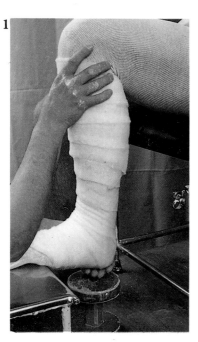 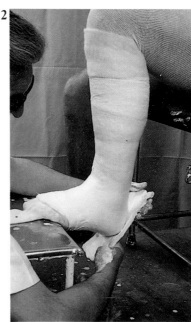 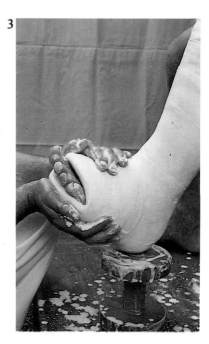

1-3   This is one of several methods of application that can be used when the ankle or foot injury is undisplaced and stable. The forefoot is supported on the edge of a firm object so that the foot is plantigrade and neither inverted or everted. The tubular gauze is applied and padding bandage is wrapped round to protect the leg, ankle and foot (**1**). 6-8 layers of plaster bandage are applied in a circular fashion. A small splint is applied to the heel and sole of the foot (**2**), the gauze is turned back to expose the toes (**3**), and the plaster is moulded around the foot and ankle. If weight bearing is intended a sole is incorporated. The patient should not take weight on the cast until the plaster is dry and hard at 24 or 48 hours; he may need crutches if he wants to mobilise immediately after the application of the cast.

26

Short leg cast: fibreglass

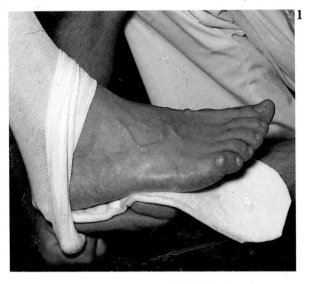

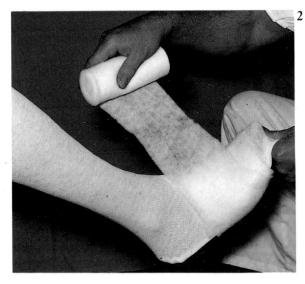

1 & 2 The patient sits or lies with his leg hanging over the end of a table. A leg stocking of tubular gauze is drawn over the leg, but between the sole and the

gauze a pad of felt is fitted [cut to shape, 0.5 - 1.0 cm (¼-½ in) thick]. Wool bandage is wrapped around the leg, foot and ankle to protect the skeletal prominences.

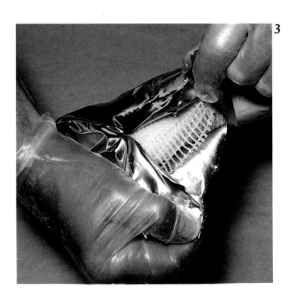

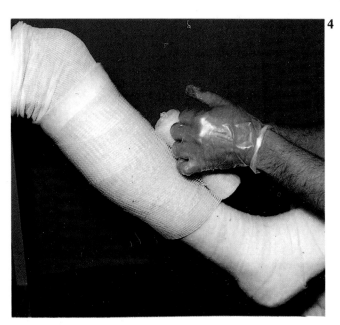

3 & 4 The operator puts on disposable gloves to protect his skin from the fibreglass bandage and opens the sealed light-proof packet. The patient's forefoot is balanced on the plasterer's knee so that the foot is plantigrade and in neutral rotation. The fibreglass bandage is wrapped around the lower leg and foot.

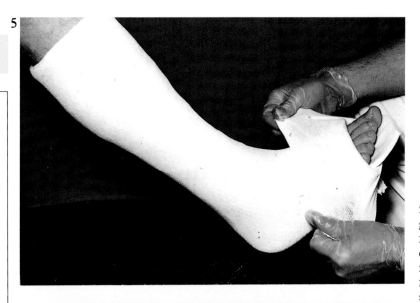

5 & 6 The top and bottom cuffs of tube gauze and padding are turned over the fibreglass to form neat smooth comfortable edges. The knee and toes are left free to move. A wet crepe bandage is wrapped firmly around the fibreglass while it is setting so that all loose edges will conform smoothly to the shape of the patient's leg.

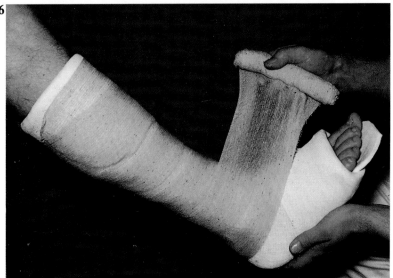

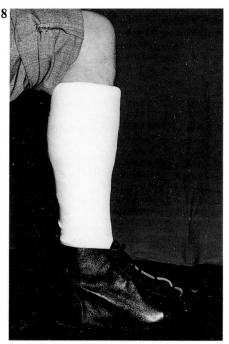

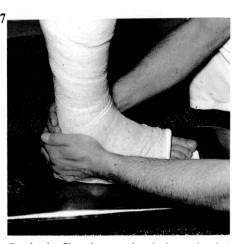

7 As the fibreglass sets hard, the patient's foot is placed on a firm horizontal surface and the cast is moulded into his heel.

8 The completed cast allows full movement of the knee and toes and is hard enough for standing and walking within 30 minutes of application. This patient is wearing a cast boot – an advantage when walking out of doors particularly in cold wet weather.

Extending a short leg cast

Extension of a short leg cast to above the knee is sometimes required to eliminate rotary stresses about the leg and ankle. Production of a Sarmiento transverse ridge and the lateral wings may provide for this (see page 34) but sometimes other injuries in the upper leg require a full thigh cast extension. This can be achieved with the patient lying down and his lower leg held elevated by an assistant (see applica-tion of a long leg cast page 39). If the injury is stable and no anaesthetic is necessary, the patient can sit on a chair with his heel on a support.

Requirements 1 roll 15 cm (6 in) padding bandage; 3 rolls 20 cm (8 in) plaster bandage; 1 splint of 20 cm (8 in) plaster bandage, 10 layers thick and 40 cm (16 in) long.

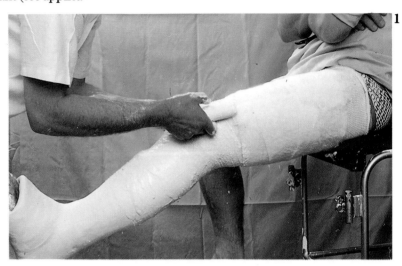

1 When the plaster is hard around the heel the patient can sit on the edge of a chair with the heel on a support. The knee must be slightly bent; this eliminates rotary stresses at a fracture site. Tubular gauze and a layer of padding bandage is applied to the thigh.

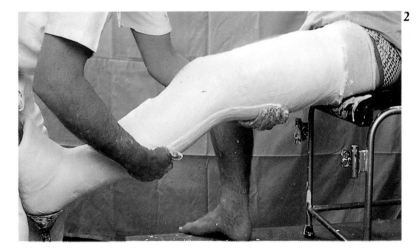

2 Plaster bandage is wrapped around the thigh with an ample overlap at the knee. The splint is added behind the knee for extra strength at this potentially weak point.

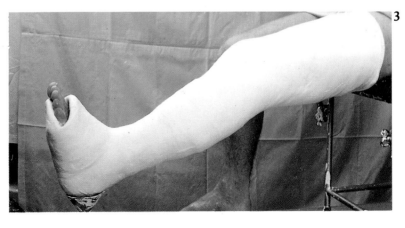

3 The top edge of padding and gauze is turned over and a final roll of plaster bandage is wrapped around the thigh and knee to give a smooth surface. The toes are free, the foot is plantigrade and the knee is slightly flexed.

Cast braces

Hinged weight bearing cast braces are a recent development in the treatment of femoral and tibial fractures. They can be applied 2 - 6 weeks after injury when the fracture is beginning to unite. Their value lies in allowing patients to walk with mobile knees and/or ankles thus leaving hospital at an earlier date. Fractures of the upper two thirds of the femoral shaft require a quadrilateral socket with or without a pelvic band, but this is not necessary for fractures of the lower femur, tibial condyles or tibial shaft. The fitting of an ankle hinge increases the patient's mobility if there is no associated injury near the ankle or foot. Cast braces can be constructed with plaster of Paris and metal hinges or with modern resin materials and plastic hinges. The latter arrangement will give a very light cast brace suitable for old and frail patients. Metal hinges give excellent support around the knee but their placement must be accurate and bending action perfect. The application of a quadrilateral socket and metal hinges is not illustrated here.

Requirements 1 special close woven elastic stocking of correct size; 20 cm (8 in) tubular gauze; 1 roll 10 cm (4 in) padding bandage; 6 rolls 10 cm (4 in) fibreglass/resin bandage; 2 hinges; 2 malleable metal bands; 1 screwdriver; 1 sponge plastic sole piece.

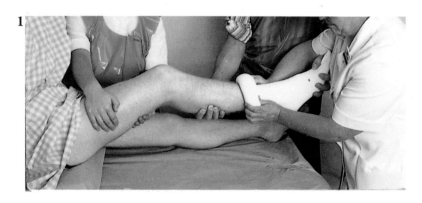

1 This patient had an undisplaced fracture of the medial tibial condyle 1 week previously. His leg is supported by 2 assistants while the special elastic stocking is applied. This is made in various sizes to fit all shapes of leg. It is firm enough to limit swelling around the knee.

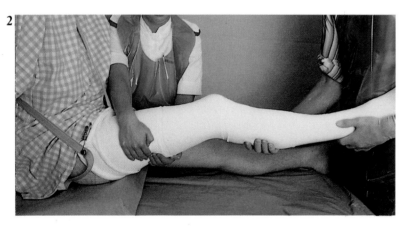

2 A second short piece of tubular gauze is added around the knee. This is used to give a smooth edge to the casts above and below the knee. A layer of padding is wrapped around the upper and lower ends of the femur and tibia to act as a protection at the margins of the cast components.

3 Resin bandages are used to form a thigh cylinder and a below knee cast including the foot. The second tubular gauze layer is cut circumferentially around the knee and folded back. The centre of the patella is marked as well as the upper edge of the tibia both medially and laterally.

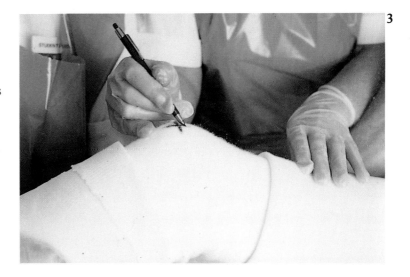

4 Using the marks as guides, plastic hinges are bent to fit the patient's leg and are temporarily held in place by the assistants. If metal hinges are to be used they are bent to fit at this stage.

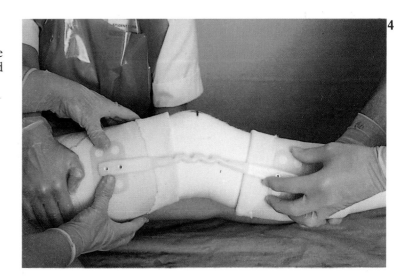

5 Malleable metal bands which can be adjusted with a screwdriver are used to hold the hinges in place while they are bound to the thigh and leg casts with resin bandages.

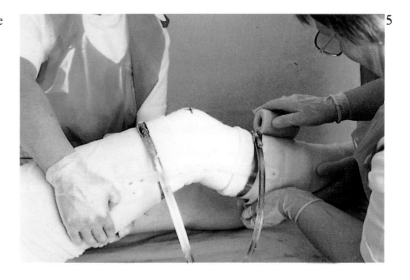

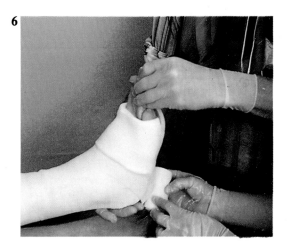

6 The toe piece of the underlying stocking is cut off and the stocking folded back to make a neat edge. A plastic foot piece is applied using more resin bandage.

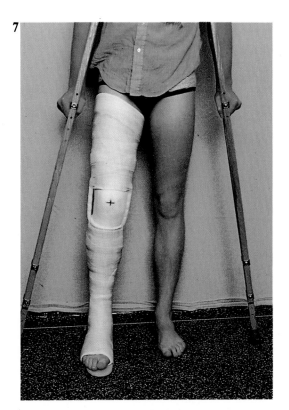

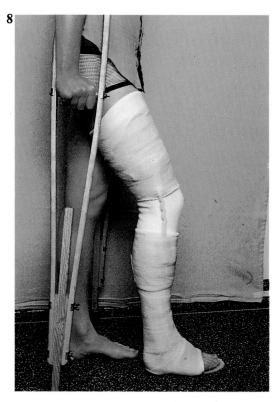

7 & 8 The modern synthetic bandages harden enough to take some weight within 30 minutes of application. Plaster of Paris requires 48 hours to reach maximum strength. This patient's cast brace allows freedom for toe movement (with the foot plantigrade) and knee flexion. The thigh is supported up to the groin and the site of injury at the knee is freed from most of the stresses of weight bearing.

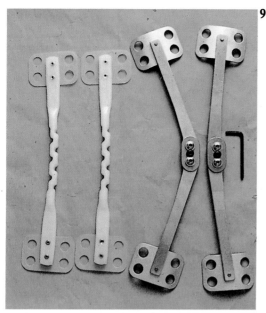

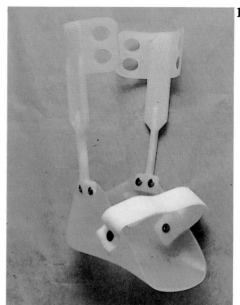

9 Plastic and metal hinges for cast braces. The shafts of metal hinges are bent to fit the contours of the knee and a jig is needed to hold them accurately in place while they are being bound to the thigh and shin casts. They are much more rigid than plastic hinges.

10 An ankle/foot piece of plastic which can be fitted to a leg cast to allow ankle movement. These are made in several sizes.

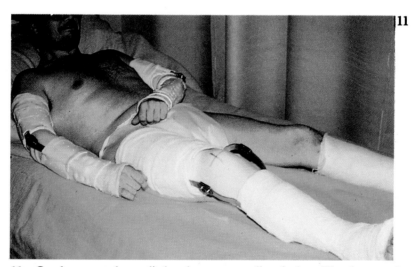

11 Cast braces can be applied to the arms as well as the legs. They increase the patient's mobility and decrease his time in hospital. This hang glider pilot who broke all four limbs would have been much more heavily dependent on nursing care without movement in his elbows and right knee.

Sarmiento cast: fibreglass

This below knee weight relieving plaster can be used for fractures of the lower leg or ankle. The weight is borne on the patellar ligament below the patella, thus unloading the fracture site. Application requires careful attention to detail particularly in fashioning the transverse ridge for the patellar ligament and the lateral wings at the knee. These wings prevent rotation of the lower leg and foot but allow full knee flexion. This type of plaster cast can be used from the beginning in fractures that are not displaced or shortened, but more usually it is applied at 2 - 4 weeks after a fracture when most of the swelling has subsided and the fracture is becoming firm. A hinged plastic foot piece can be incorporated to allow ankle movement. Sarmiento casts can be made of plaster of Paris, or with resinous or fibreglass bandages (as illustrated). These are light, durable, and waterproof but expensive.

Requirements: 1 leg stocking of tubular gauze; 1 roll of fibreglass bandage 3.6 m (4 yards) × 10 cm (4 in); 2 rolls of fibreglass bandage 3.6 m (4 yards) × 15 cm (6 in); 1 roll of crepe bandage 3 m (3 yards) × 15 cm (6 in) wide; gloves.

If plaster is used the following will be required: 2 rolls of 10 cm (4 in) padding bandage; 6 - 8 rolls of 15 cm (6 in) plaster bandage; 1 piece of felt 1.0 cm (½ in) thick for making a sole.

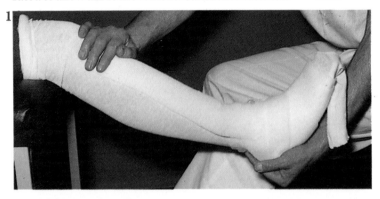

1 The patient lies or sits on a table with his legs hanging over one end. An assistant is required to support and steady the fracture site and knee. The felt sole is held in place while the tubular gauze leg stocking is fitted.

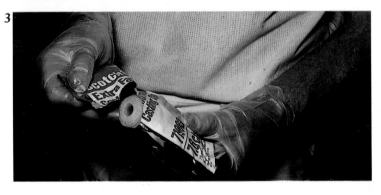

2 A strip of wool bandage is laid up the front of the leg and additional padding is wrapped around below the knee and around the foot and ankle (this pads the sharp edge of the tibia).

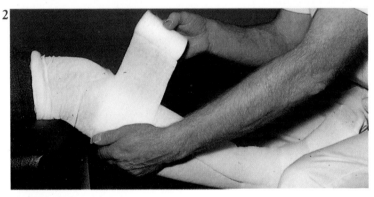

3 The operator, wearing disposable gloves to protect his skin, opens a sealed packet of fibreglass bandage.

MEDICAL ECONOMICS BOOKS
P.O. BOX C-779
BROOKLYN, N.Y. 11205-9066

INVOICE DATE
10-30-86

ACCOUNT MULTI
96993-

INVOICE NO. T
42966 0

S D A ZORN MD
O 1301 HODGES DR
L TALLAHASSEE FL
D
T
O

32308

LOC. BAT. PAYMENT
1FL 06 27.95

SHIP VIA
U.P.S.

TITLE NO.	DESCRIPTION	SYM.	QUANT.	PRICE	AMOUNT
04239	MILLS/CA PLAST TECHN		1	25.95 000	25.95
	PREPAID				

THIS IS NOT A BILL

THANK YOU

A/T A KEY PDRZ6

WEIGHT

BOOKS TOTAL	25.95
SALES TAX	.
27.95 POST/HANDLING	2.00
TOTAL AMOUNT	27.95

ZONE
5

PACKING SLIP

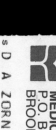

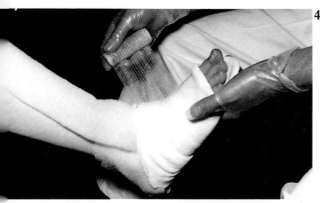

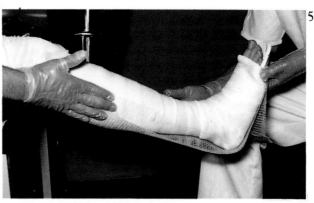

4 The 10 cm bandage is wrapped firmly around the foot. It is deceptively thin and fragile at first but quickly sets into a very strong cast even if only 3 layers thick.

5 The remainder of this bandage is used to make a double layer splint up the back of the leg. The assistant holds the top edge of the splint. One 15 cm (6 in) fibreglass bandage is used to complete the cast as far as the tibial tubercle, wrapping it firmly around the leg.

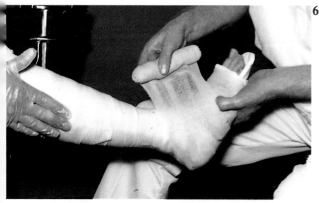

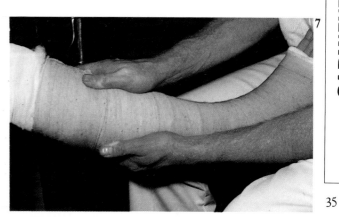

6 A wet crepe bandage is applied on top of the fibreglass while setting occurs.

7 The loose edges are held in place to conform exactly with the contours of the leg.

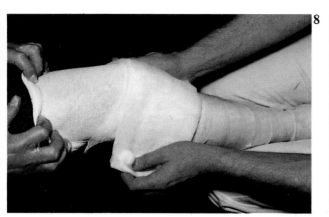

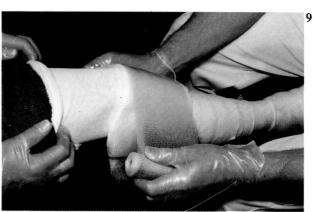

8 The cotton bandage is removed and additional padding is applied around the knee. The assistant pulls the gauze stocking upwards over the thigh.

9 The second 15 cm (6 in) roll of fibreglass bandage is used to form a transverse splint at the level of the knee but adhering to the top of the plaster cylinder.

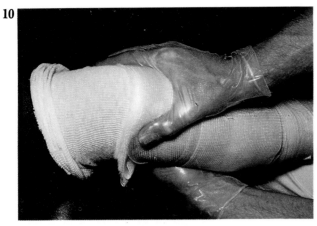

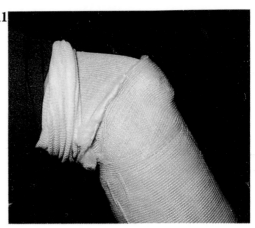

10 As the splint sets the transverse ridge is formed at the level of the patellar ligament by the pressure of the manipulator's hand.

11 The transverse ridge with wings extending on either side of the knee prevents rotation. The back of the knee is left free to allow full flexion.

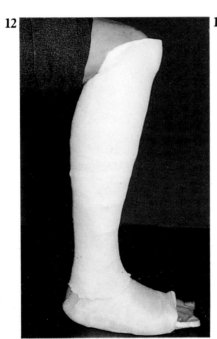

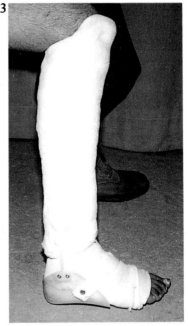

12 The tubular gauze is turned down to make a neat top edge. The cast will be dry enough for weight bearing after 30 minutes.

13 A Sarmiento cast made from plaster of Paris with a plastic ankle hinge and a plastic sole plate.

Knee cylinder cast

This type of plaster is used for injuries and operations around the knee. It leaves the hip, ankle and foot quite mobile. The knee is usually fixed in a position of extension. When the patient stands up the weight of the plaster is supported by the lower leg around the ankle; consequently good padding above the malleoli is required to prevent skin ulceration. Subsequent swelling can impede the circulation of the foot. This can be avoided by applying adhesive supportive strapping to the foot, ankle and lower leg.

Requirements Leg stocking of tubular gauze; 2 rolls of 15 cm (6 in) wool bandage; 1 strip of adhesive felt [4 cm (1½ in) wide × 0.5 cm (¼ in) thick × girth of ankle]; 4 rolls of 20 cm (8 in) plaster bandage; 1 splint of 15 cm (6 in) plaster bandage (5 layers thick × length between mid thigh and mid calf).

1 A leg stocking of tubular gauze is applied to the leg. Adhesive elastic tape is applied around the foot, ankle, and lower leg to prevent later swelling when the patient starts walking. If the patient is allergic to adhesives, 2 layers of elastic tubular gauze or a crepe bandage can be used. The length of the patient's leg is measured from mid calf to mid thigh and a 5 layer plaster splint is cut to length from 15 cm (6 in) plaster bandage.

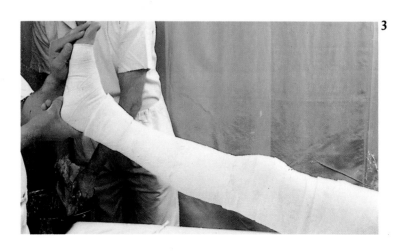

2 A band of adhesive felt is firmly taped around the ankle malleoli to protect the skin from the plaster cylinder which slides down the leg when the patient stands up.

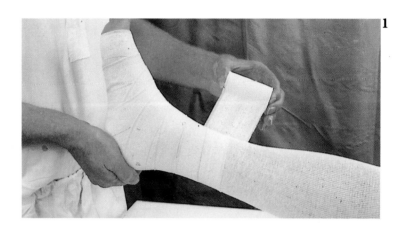

3 An assistant holds the leg elevated as a wool bandage is wrapped around the leg. Circular turns of plaster bandage are applied to the leg with even tension. The genitalia should be protected from plaster. The plaster should extend from near the groin to within 1 cm (½ in) of the lower edge of the adhesive felt at the ankle.

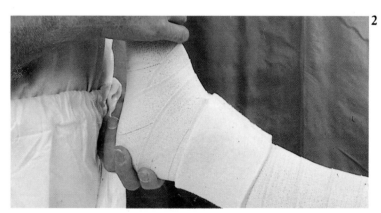

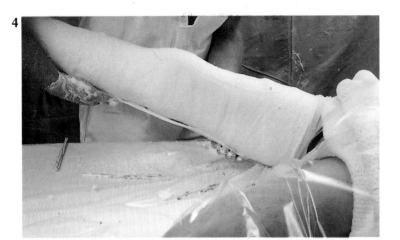

4 The plaster splint is applied behind the knee to strengthen the cast. Further rolls of plaster bandage are wrapped round the leg to give a cylinder of even thickness.

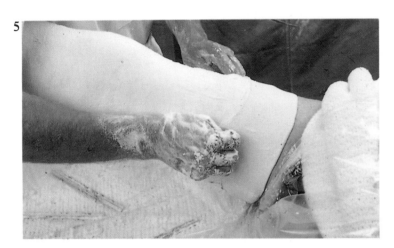

5 The gauze and padding are turned over at the upper margin of the cylinder to give a comfortable smooth edge at the groin. As the plaster hardens the surgeon can give a few degrees of flexion at the knee or can produce a valgus or varus stress as the case requires.

38

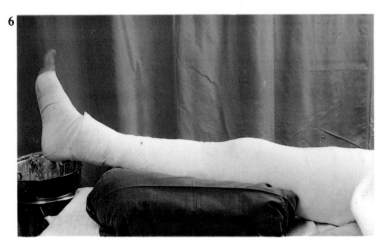

6 The completed cylinder cast is allowed to harden for a few hours on a pillow before the patient is mobilised.

Long leg cast

Long leg casts are applied to immobilise fractures or to support operations on the lower leg and ankle. They are not effective for immobilising the thigh (if this is required a hip spica or a cast brace should be applied) and only applicable to some injuries and operations at the lower femur to upper tibia. A few degrees of knee flexion will prevent any rotatory movements being transmitted to a fracture site in the lower leg. This enables the patient to turn over in bed without pain and renders accidental jerks to the forefoot relatively painless. There are several methods of application of a long leg cast, only one of which is illustrated. This patient, with a fracture of the tibia and fibula, is supine and anaesthetised. Patients with undisplaced fractures frequently do not need any anaesthesia.

Requirements Leg stocking of tubular gauze; 2 - 3 rolls of 10 or 15 cm (4 or 6 in) wool bandage; 8 - 10 rolls of 15 or 20 cm (6 or 8 in) plaster bandage.

1-4 The thigh is supported by one assistant and traction is applied to the foot and ankle by a second assistant who also gives additional support to the fracture site (**1**). Tubular gauze and wool bandage are applied to the lower leg and a plaster cylinder is applied between the knee and ankle. As it sets, the fracture site is supported by the surgeon to correct angulation and rotation deformities (**2**). With the first assistant still supporting the thigh, the second assistant uses one hand to support the fracture site and the other hand to grip the toes while the plaster dries with the foot in the neutral position (**3**). The second assistant then holds the leg with both hands with the foot against his chest. In this position he can comfortably control knee flexion and rotation of the lower leg (**4**). Hip flexion and abduction will allow padding and plaster bandage to be applied to the knee and thigh. The tubular gauze is turned back in the groin and at the ankle to ensure a smooth finish. The toes are allowed a full range of movement.

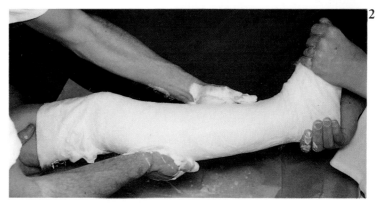

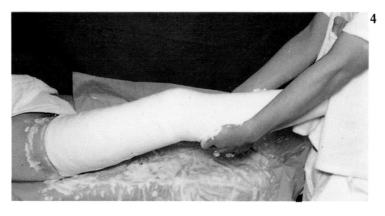

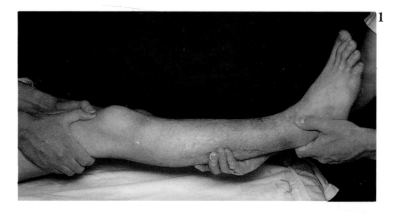

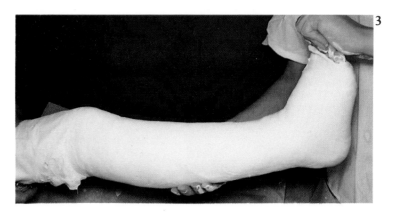

Sole construction

Plaster of Paris must be at least 1 cm (½ in) thick on the sole of a leg cast when it has dried out completely to take the weight of the patient when walking. If the plaster becomes wet from sweat, bathing, or rain, it will soften and disintegrate. Consequently a strong sole is required, often with a shock absorbing material incorporated such as sponge rubber, plastic or felt. A variety of proprietary rubber or metal soles and heels are available to add to the bottom of a cast. Patients must be fully instructed in the care of their cast and must be warned not to bear weight (if this is intended) until the plaster has fully dried out. Crutches may be required until then. Fibreglass or resin casts do not require so long to harden, usually 30 - 60 minutes suffices. These casts do not disintegrate if wet. However, the sole still requires to be considerably thicker than the rest of the cast. Whatever type of cast or sole is applied it is an advantage to the patient to wear a cast boot to protect the toes and to keep the foot dry and warm.

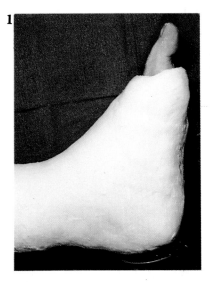

1 It may be sufficient to have no more than a very thick layer of plaster if the patient is to undertake only partial weight bearing with the aid of crutches. A cast boot may also be worn.

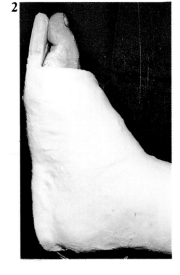

2 A leg cast with a compressible plastic sole plate incorporated. This projects forward to protect the plantar surface of the toes. A cast boot will give additional protection.

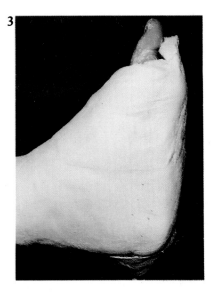

3 A leg cast with a piece of felt as a shock absorber. A cast boot is also required for walking out of doors.

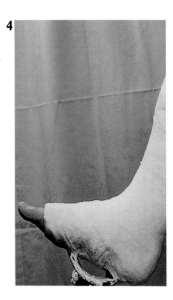

4 A leg cast with a proprietary metal hoop as a soleplate. This is strong and durable so that no cast boot is required when walking out of doors. However, the toes and cast need protection from cold and rain by the use of a thick bandage or sock.

Hip spica

This large plaster may be used to immobilise injuries or support operative procedures around the pelvis, the hip joint or the upper end of the femur. It must take purchase on the lower ribs and extend at least as far as just above the knee on the affected side. A cast that ends below the ribs allows movement at the hip and cuts into the abdomen uncomfortably. If there are injuries, operative procedures or weakness below the knee, the cast must be extended to include the lower leg and often the foot and ankle as well. In children and others who are very mobile it is necessary to immobilise the hips on both sides. Usually the cast extends lower down the leg on the affected side. Hip spica casts are heavy and cumbersome so that walking with crutches (only possible if one hip is free) can be slow and tiring. The perineal region must be left free for toilet purposes but it is not possible for the patient to use a conventional toilet even if he is able to move himself about. Consequently, he needs help with his toilet until the cast can be removed. The edges of the dry plaster can be protected from soiling by waterproof adhesive tape.

Requirements Body stocking and leg stocking of tubular gauze; Adhesive felt [0.5 cm (¼ in) thick]; 6 rolls 15 cm (6 in) wool bandage; 10 rolls 20 cm (8 in) plaster bandage; 3 - 4 splints [5 layers × body girth × 15 or 20 cm (6 or 8 in)]; 3 splints [10 layers × nipple to knee length × 20 cm (8 in)].

1   The cast is applied with the patient lying on an orthopaedic table. This consists of supports for the shoulders, the sacrum and the feet with infinite adjustability of all 4 components. The sacral support and the perineal post require padding for comfort. Usually the patient is anaesthetised. The trunk girth is measured in order to prepare 3 - 4 splints [5 layers × 20 cm (8 in) × body girth]. The distance from nipple to knee is also measured to prepare 3 splints [20 cm (8 in) plaster bandage 10 layers] thick of this length.

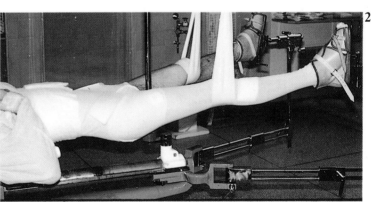

2   The patient is placed on the orthopaedic table with his arms supported to achieve complete clearance of the lower ribs. A body stocking is applied over the head and pulled down to cover the lower trunk and pelvis. The leg is also covered by tubular bandage.

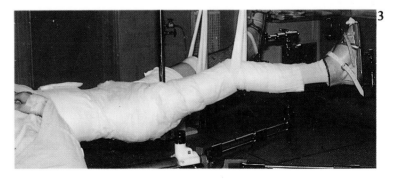

3   The desired position of the hips, knees and feet are now adjusted by the surgeon. Pads of adhesive felt are cut to size to protect the iliac crests anteriorly and the spinous processes posteriorly.

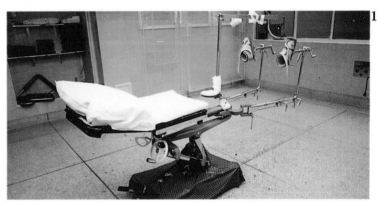

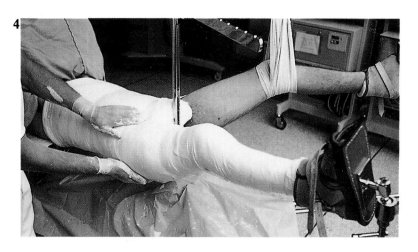

4 The trunk is encircled by several layers of 20 cm (8 in) plaster bandage. These layers are smoothed down and any air bubbles removed.

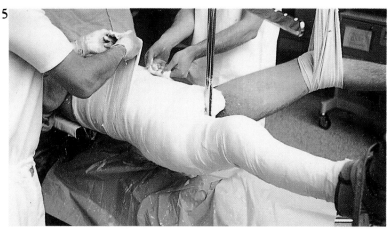

5 The trunk part of the cast is strengthened by 3 or 4 overlapping circumferential splints, previously prepared. These are smoothed in to place and all air bubbles removed. The leg is encircled by turns of 20 cm (8 in) plaster bandage. The three long splints also previously prepared are applied lengthwise on the front, the side and at the back of the hip from the lower ribs to the knee.

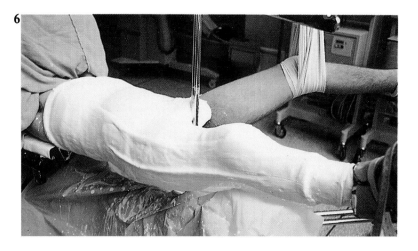

6 The lateral splint is 'ridged' or 'girdered' to give extra strength. The back of the hip is always the weak point in this plaster cast.

7   In the majority of cases the knee is fixed in a position of slight flexion (after removal of the suspension bandage) with a few turns of 20 cm (8 in) plaster bandage. In this case the lower leg is released and suspended from the toes by an assistant and enclosed in plaster with the foot plantigrade and in neutral inversion/eversion. The top and bottom margins of the tubular gauze are turned back to give a smooth edge at the toes and round the chest. The margin of the plaster at the groin should be high enough to give full flexion of the free hip.

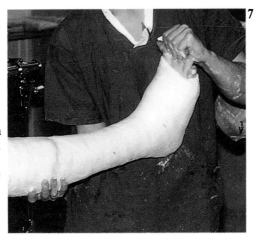

8   While the cast is being applied it is of advantage to have the patient's bed prepared with several pillows laid transversely. This will prevent the wet plaster from being deformed by the weight of the patient's body against a hard mattress.

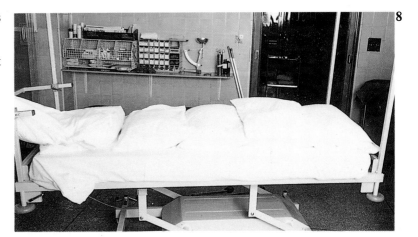

9   Once on his bed, the patient can be turned on to his face every 2 hours or so to allow the posterior surfaces of the plaster to dry. When the plaster is completely dry (2-3 days) the perineal margins can be protected from faecal soiling by trimming and applying waterproof adhesive tape.

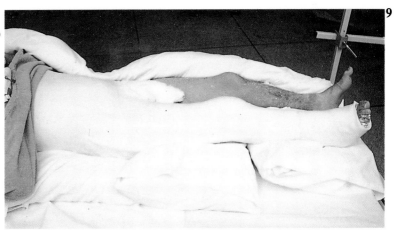

Children's hip casts

Children who have operations or injuries around the hips usually require some form of splintage. This may take the form of a unilateral or bilateral hip spica cast or bilateral leg cylinders joined by a cross bar. Small infants usually have such mobile joints that bilateral hip spica casts are needed to achieve complete immobilisation of the affected joint. The perineum is left widely exposed for toilet purposes.

Bilateral leg cylinders are easily adjusted by the application of a cross bar to give what ever hip position may be needed.

Requirements Body and leg stockings of tubular gauze; 1 - 2 rolls of 10 cm (4 in) wool bandage; 6 - 10 rolls of 10 cm (4 in) plaster bandage; A short piece of wood.

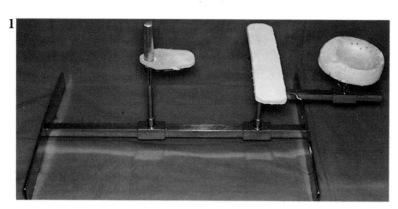

1 An orthopaedic frame to support infants and small children when they are having hip or leg casts applied. It is readily adjustable to support different body sizes. It consists of a perineal post, pelvic support, shoulder cross bar and saucer-like head support. The pelvic support and perineal post require padding to avoid pressure sores.

2 The infant is placed on the frame and the supports adjusted. The anaesthetist and assistants control the position of the head and arms. The surgeon places the legs and hips in the position he requires – in this instance in full abduction and internal rotation.

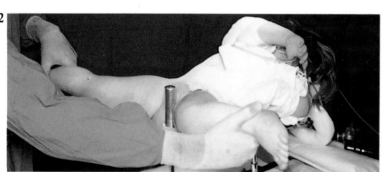

3 Both assistants now take the legs to maintain the required position while body and legs stockings are applied and/ or wool bandages are wrapped around the trunk and legs. A cross bar of thin wood is selected and cut to size. The trunk and legs are now encircled by plaster bandages [usually 10 cm (4 in), sometimes 15 cm (6 in) for bigger children].

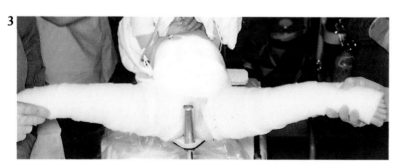

4 The cross bar is covered in plaster bandage and fitted to the legs at knee or shin level. The feet are incorporated in the plaster in neutral position.

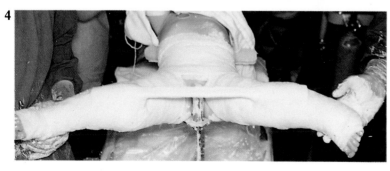

5 This child's hips are being splinted in flexion, abduction and external rotation after surgery. The orthopaedic frame is not required, provided the child's trunk is supported by one or two pillows. The perineum is protected by padding, leg stockings are drawn on and the size of the cross bar selected. Wool bandage is then wrapped around the legs.

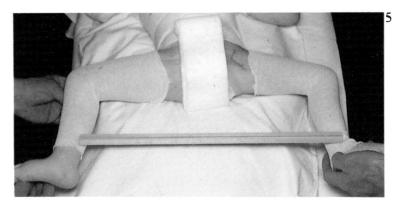

6 Plaster bandages are applied to form leg cylinders with the knees flexed. An ample cuff of gauze stocking and padding above and below is left free of plaster. The cross bar is wrapped in plaster bandage and is applied just above the ankles.

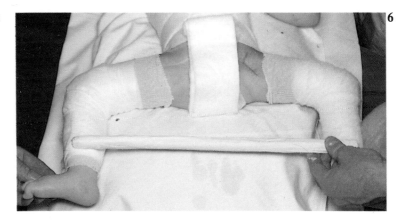

7 The cuffs of stocking and padding are turned over to give smooth edges at the top and bottom margins of the plasters. The feet and ankles are allowed freedom.

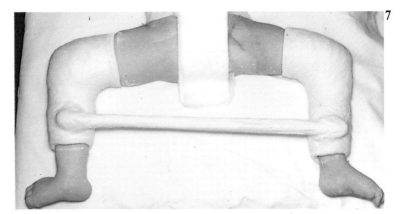

45

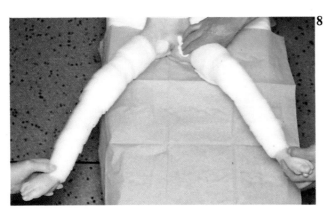

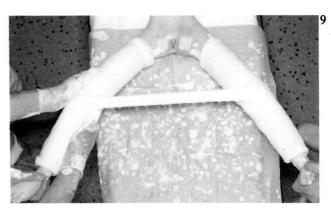

8 This child's hips have undergone surgery but will be stable in abduction and neutral rotation. The child's trunk is supported on pillows and the legs wrapped in wool bandage.

9 Plaster cylinders are applied to the legs and a suitable cross bar incorporated at knee level. This maintains the position of the hips while healing takes place.

Lumbar jacket

Lumbar plaster jackets are occasionally applied for prolapsed intervertebral discs, minor or healing fractures of the lumbar spine and as a pre-operative trial of splintage before lumbar spinal fusion. They are sometimes used for post fusion splintage as well. They must be fitted with the patient upright, either sitting, or, preferably, standing. Removable plastic jackets, made from heat malleable plastics, are gradually replacing plaster jackets.

Requirements   Body stocking of tubular gauze; Pads of felt 0.5 cm (¼ in) thick; 3 rolls of 15 cm (6 in) wool bandage; 6 rolls of 20 cm (8 in) plaster bandage; 3 - 4 splints of 20 cm (8 in) plaster 5 layers thick × body girth.

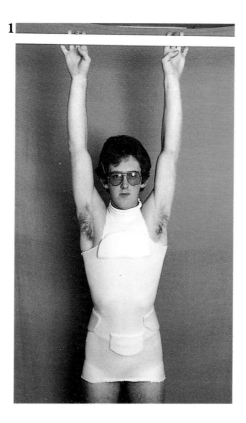
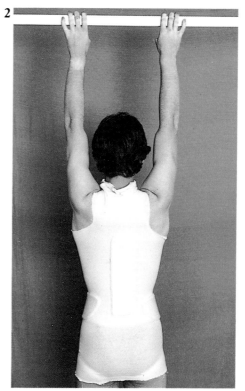

1 & 2   The plaster is best applied with the patient standing. His arms can be supported by assistants or he can hold on to a bar above his shoulder level. This will bring the lumbar spine into slight extension. A body stocking is applied with holes cut for the arms. The girth of the trunk is measured and 3 or 4 splints of plaster of this length are prepared [20 cm (8 in) wide and 5 layers thick]. The bony prominences are padded by adhesive felt over the sternum, pubis, the iliac crests and the spinous processes of the lumbar and lower thoracic vertebrae. These are cut to size and the edges bevelled with scissors.

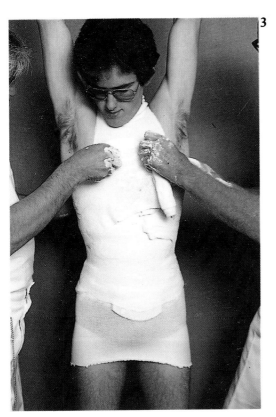

3 The first layers of plaster are applied by 3 circular turns of 20 cm bandages.

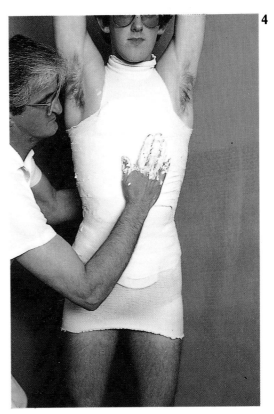

4 The initial layers of plaster are smoothed and contoured to the shape of the trunk. All bubbles must be eliminated.

47

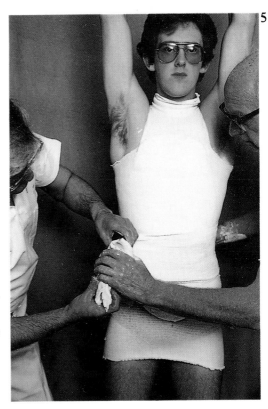

5 The previously prepared splints are dipped in water and applied horizontally around the trunk starting at the bottom. It is best to have two assistants applying these, each holding one end of the splint. The splints should overlap by 1 - 2 cm (½ - ¾ in) and should be contoured to the curvatures of the upper and lower margins of the jacket.

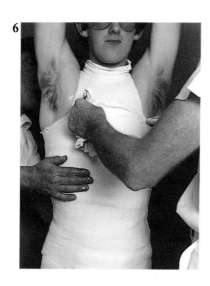

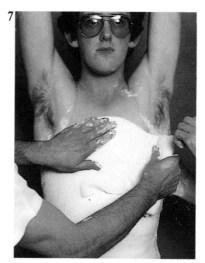

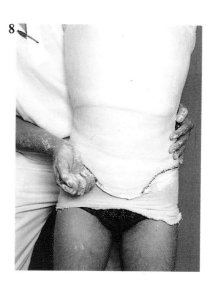

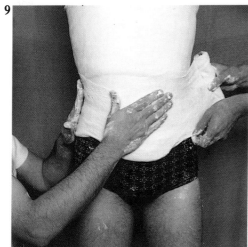

6-9 The splints are smoothed down on the underlying layers, eliminating air bubbles (**6**). The upper margin of the plaster should be highest in the front over the manubriosternal joint (**7**) and lowest at the back, level with the inferior angles of the scapulae. The lower margins should be lowest over the pubis and clear of the groin to allow full flexion of the hips (**8**). 2 or 3 circular bandages are finally applied to provide a smooth surface to the jacket (**9**).

48

10 The body stocking is trimmed to leave a layer of stocking protruding 5 cm (2 in) above and below the plaster jacket. This is turned over and incorporated below the last application of plaster bandage to make a neat finish. A circular hole can be cut out over the abdomen if the patient's girth is likely to increase markedly at meal times or if breathing is mainly diaphragmatic.

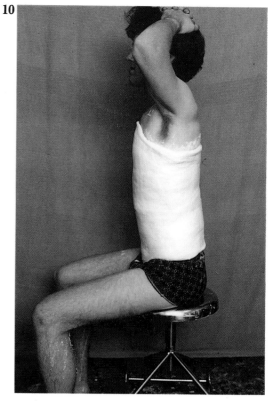

Finger strapping

Undisplaced stable fractures of the proximal and middle phalanges can be successfully treated by splinting the injured finger to the adjoining uninjured finger. This allows movement at all the finger joints and helps to prevent joint stiffness. A number of techniques are available, three of which are illustrated here.

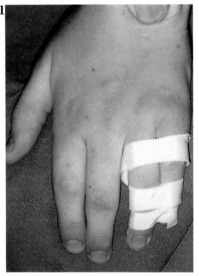

1 This patient had an undisplaced fracture of the middle phalanx of the ring finger. Strips of adhesive tape 1 cm (½ in) wide encircle the proximal, middle and terminal phalanges of the ring and little fingers, allowing freedom of movement of the interphalangeal joints.

2 In this patient an undisplaced fracture of the proximal phalanx of the index finger has been splinted against the uninjured long finger. Care must be taken not to apply the tape too tightly, especially elastic tape. A strip of padding is placed between the fingers.

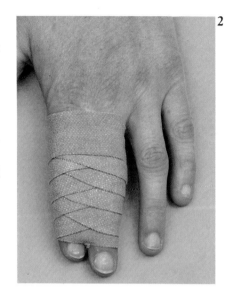

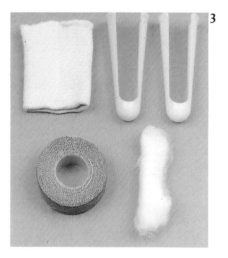

3-5 Alternative splintage of adjacent fingers for stable undisplaced fractures of the middle and terminal phalanges using two removable plastic shells with custom made elastic cotton cylinders which are joined together (**3**). The elastic cotton cylinders are applied over the plastic shells which are then withdrawn (**4**). This splintage allows some movement at the interphalangeal joints (**5**). The elastic cotton splints can be removed very easily.

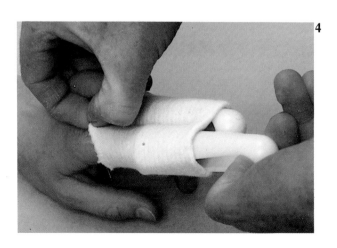

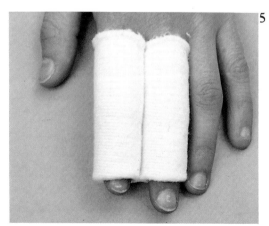

Finger casts: Boxer's fracture

This type of boxer's fracture is found at the neck of the fifth metacarpal. The knuckle joint is recessed and angled but can be reduced in most cases by flexing the proximal joints of the little finger and using the proximal phalanx to push back the head of the metacarpal. Not every fracture requires treatment and of those that do some can be fixed by the application of screws or pins. Many are treated symptomatically by application of elastic adhesive tape.

Requirements   1 roll of 10 cm (4 in) wool bandage; 2 rolls of 10 cm (4 in) plaster bandage.

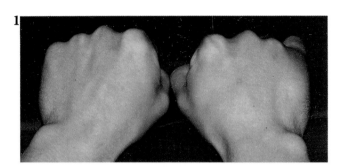

1   Recession of the knuckle on the ulnar side of the right hand from a fracture of the fifth metacarpal neck.

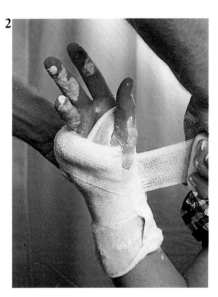
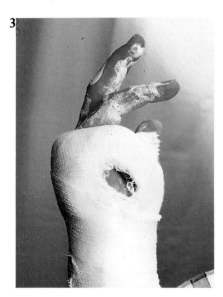

2 & 3   Under regional or general anaesthesia the fifth finger is flexed across the palm – so that it points to the base of the thumb. This gives the correct rotation. The hand is protected by a layer of padding. A roll of plaster bandage is applied to support the wrist and fifth finger. The fifth proximal phalanx is pushed backwards on the metacarpal and the wet plaster is moulded to hold the reduction. The hole at the side allows observation of the circulation to the finger.

Finger casts for unstable proximal and middle phalangeal fractures

Unstable fractures of the proximal and middle phalanges tend to angulate and shorten under the influence of the strong flexor tendons. They can be reduced under regional or general anaesthetic and held by a plaster or metal splintage or a combination as demonstrated here.

Requirements   1 roll of 10 cm (4 in) wool bandage; 3 rolls of 10 cm (4 in) plaster bandage; 1 strip of malleable metal splint; 1 roll of 2.5 cm (1 in) elastic adhesive tape.

1   The fracture is reduced by traction.

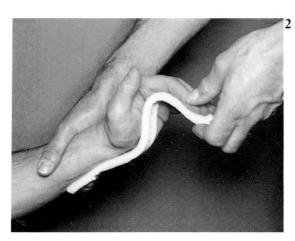

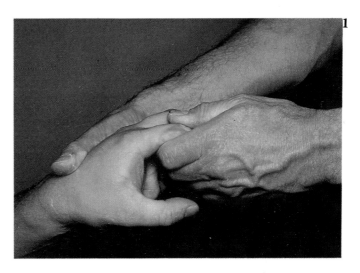

2   The semi rigid metal splint is bent to conform to the contours of the hand with the wrist slightly dorsiflexed, the metacarpophalangeal joints flexed to 90° and the interphalangeal joints slightly flexed.

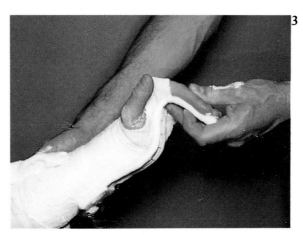

3   Padding is applied to the forearm, wrist and palm to protect the skin. Two plaster bandages are wrapped around the forearm and palm; these incorporate the malleable metal wire splint on the volar aspect of the wrist, palm and fingers.

4 The plaster is completed around the forearm, wrist and palm and a strip of padding is placed between the fractured index and adjacent long fingers.

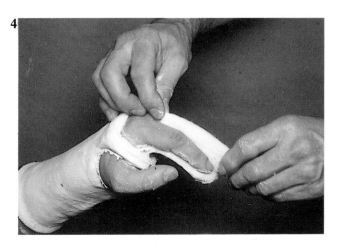

5 The fractured finger is taped to the metal splint and adjacent finger with 2.5 cm (1 in) adhesive tape without any compression.

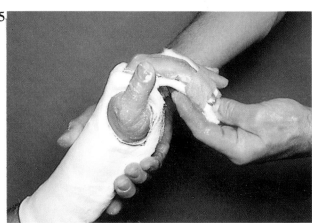

6 The metal can then be bent to achieve the final position with the metacarpophalangeal joints flexed to 90° and the interphalangeal joints slightly flexed. This demonstrates if any rotational deformity is present at the fracture site which requires correction by a second manipulation. This position avoids contracture of the collateral ligaments which causes much stiffness at the metacarpophalangeal joints.

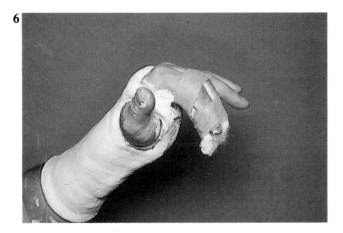

Finger casts: Mallet finger

This deformity is caused by rupture of the extensor tendon insertion on the dorsum of the terminal phalanx. The terminal phalanx is held bent by the flexor tendon and no active extension is possible. The extensor tendon will sometimes heal if the terminal joint is held extended uninterruptedly for up to 6 weeks. This can be achieved by plaster of Paris or a variety of specially made splints. The prognosis is better if a small fragment of bone is avulsed from the terminal phalanx.

Requirements A tube of 10 cm (4 in) plaster bandage 3-4 layers thick; 7.5 or 3 cm (3 or 1¼ in) bandage is used for children.

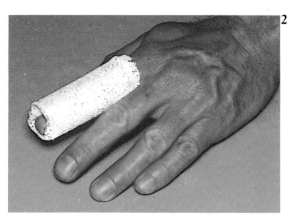

1 Splinting with plaster. The patient is shown the correct position for his finger before the plaster is applied. Thus, while it is setting he can maintain the reduced position by his own effort. The proximal interphalangeal joint should be flexed to prevent the plaster tube from falling off when set.

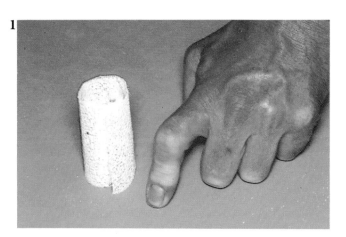

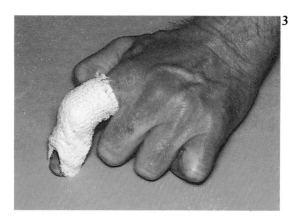

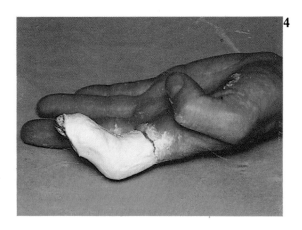

2-4 The tube of dry plaster bandage is fitted over the patient's finger (**2**). The finger is dipped in water with the tube held in place. The patient adopts the reduced position while the plaster sets hard (**3**). As the plaster hardens the terminal interphalangeal joint is held hyperextended and the proximal joint flexed (**4**). The patient is instructed to keep the plaster dry for 4-6 weeks.

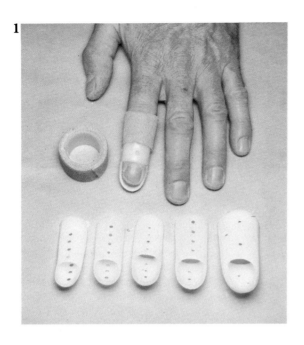

1 Plastic splints of different sizes for treating mallet fingers. These hyperextend the terminal interphalangeal joint. The correct size must be selected to obtain a comfortable fit. The splint is retained by a single layer of adhesive tape at the base. If the finger becomes wet, maceration of the skin will occur. The splint should be re-applied regularly and the skin dried. During this procedure the terminal joint must never be allowed to bend otherwise healing has to begin all over again.

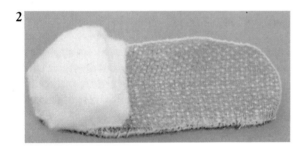

2 & 3 Simple wooden splint. Another form of mallet finger hyperextension splint can be constructed from a wooden spatula and a small piece of adhesive felt. The wooden spatula is padded by a layer of elastic adhesive tape. This spatula splint is applied with 2.5 cm (1 in) elastic adhesive tape. Regular re-application is required at intervals. Too tight an application will result in painful ischaemia.

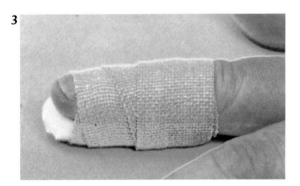

Thumb strapping

Sprains of the two joints of the thumb and fractures of the thumb that have reached an advanced state of healing can be supported by applying elastic adhesive tape 2.5 cm (1 inch) wide. The patient should be questioned about any skin allergies to adhesive tape before application.

Requirements   1 roll of adhesive tape 2.5 × 150 cm (1 × 60 in).

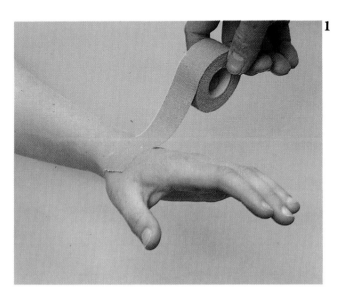

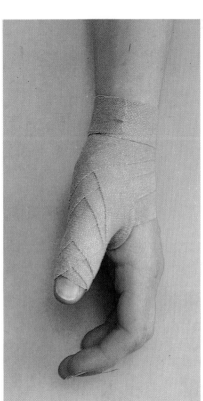

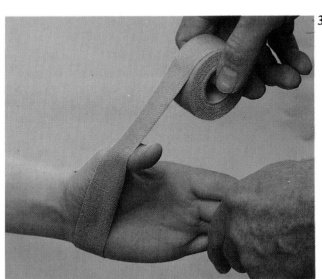

1-3   The tape is applied first across the wrist and then wound around the thumb and back across the wrist in an overlapping figure of eight. Care must be taken not to apply the tape with too much tension (especially with elastic tape) as this will cause ischaemia with subsequent pain and swelling. The final configuration firmly supports the thumb.

Thumb casts: dorsal splint (slab)

Stable fractures of the shaft of the 1st metacarpal and the proximal phalanx of the thumb can be splinted by a dorsal splint (slab) which extends from the wrist to the tip of the thumb. A larger plaster would unnecessarily interfere with the use of the forearm and the palm.

Requirements Tubular gauze; 1 roll of 10 cm (4 in) wool bandage; 1 splint 5 layers 20 × 15 cm (8 × 6 in).

56

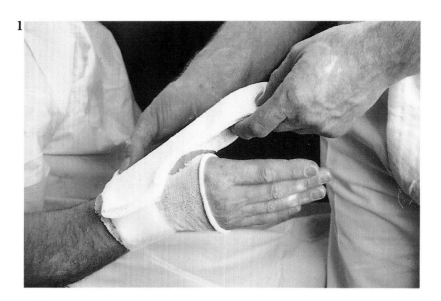

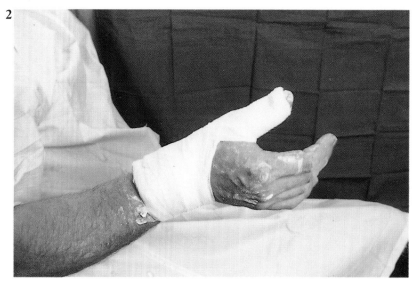

1 & 2 The plaster splint is prepared with 5 layers of 15 cm (6 in) wide bandage about 20 cm (8 in) long. It is narrowed at one end by cutting off the shoulders of the splint to fit three quarters of the circumference. The plaster splint is moulded around the thumb and wrist and held in place by a cotton bandage.

Thumb casts: Bennetts' fracture

A Bennetts' fracture dislocation occurs at the base of the thumb, usually by a blow on the clenched fist. The thumb is shortened at the fracture site by the pull of the attached tendons. It is lengthened to normality by pulling and this lengthened position has to be retained by abduction of the thumb and moulding of the plaster. A good reduction is often impossible to attain by manipulation and an operation may be required.

Requirements   Tubular gauze; 1 roll 10 cm (4 in) plaster bandage.

Small felt pads over the dorsum of the first metacarpal base and anterior to first metacarpal head.

1   Under regional or general anaesthetic the manipulator pulls the thumb out to length, usually with some abduction of the thumb as well.

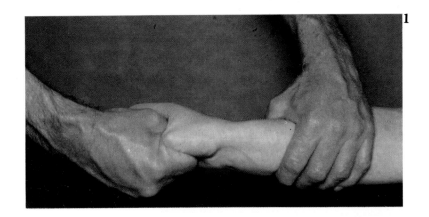

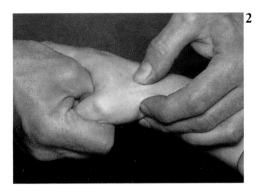

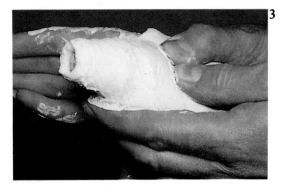

2   The fracture is reduced by the manipulator applying thumb and finger pressure at the base of the 1st metacarpal. Tube gauze is applied to the thumb and forearm with the felt pads pressed into place at either end of the first metacarpal i.e. anterior to the metacarpal head and posterior to the metacarpal base. A covering of padding around the thumb and wrist is added. Plaster of Paris bandages [3 or 4 × 10 cm (4 in)] are used to encircle the thumb and forearm.

3   As the plaster sets the manipulator presses into the base of the first metacarpal with abduction and extension of the thumb to maintain reduction of the fracture.

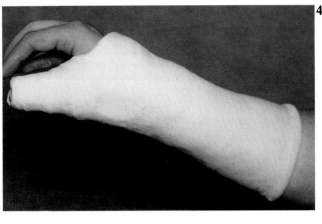

4   The completed plaster extends from the tip of the thumb to below the elbow. The wrist is slightly dorsiflexed.

Scaphoid cast

Scaphoid casts are applied to hold fractures of the scaphoid and some fractures at the base of the thumb. They are similar to short arm casts but also immobilise the thumb. In the majority of cases they can be applied without a general anaesthetic and often without an assistant if the patient is co-operative. Scaphoid fractures are usually not displaced and do not require reduction.

Requirements Tubular gauze; 1 roll 10 cm (4 in) wool bandage; 3 rolls 10 cm (4 in) plaster bandage.

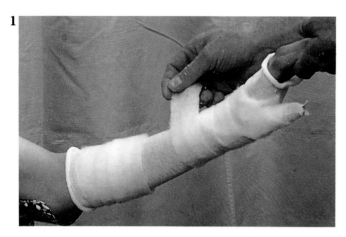

1 The patient is asked to hold his hand as if he were grasping a glass, i.e. with the forearm in neutral rotation, the wrist in slight dorsiflexion and the thumb semi-opposed. Padding is required to protect the hairs and skeletal prominences but an unpadded cast can be applied after 2 weeks if the first cast becomes loose.

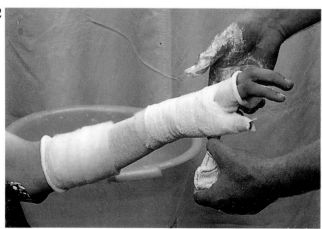

2 The plaster should immobilise the metacarpophalangeal joint of the thumb as well as the wrist. The terminal interphalangeal joint of the thumb is not immobilised unless there is additional damage in this region.

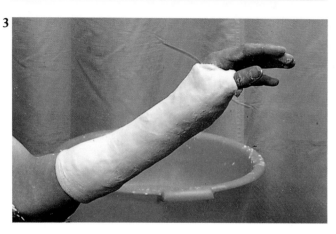

3 The completed plaster allows complete freedom to the elbow, knuckles and terminal joint of the thumb. As the plaster sets, final moulding of the wrist and thumb position is possible. The patient should demonstrate his ability to oppose the thumb to index and long fingers. If the patient cannot put his plastered arm down the sleeve of his jacket he is unlikely to be able to perform a pinch and the plaster has been wrongly applied.

Short arm cast

Short arm casts are frequently used for fractures around the wrist. They extend from knuckles to elbow and usually leave the elbow, thumb and fingers completely free. The wrist may be fixed in a dorsiflexed or palmar flexed position depending on the nature of the fracture. It is not possible to maintain a full supination (palm up) or pronation (palm down) position with a short arm cast – additional splintage of a flexed elbow is required in this case.

Requirements Tubular gauze; 1 roll of 10 cm (4 in) wool bandage; 3 rolls of 10 cm (4 in) plaster bandage.

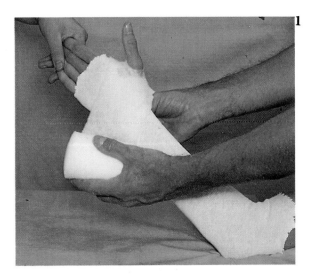

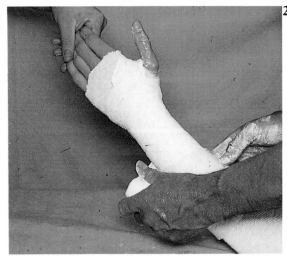

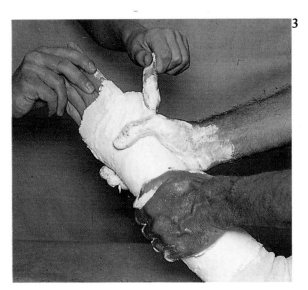

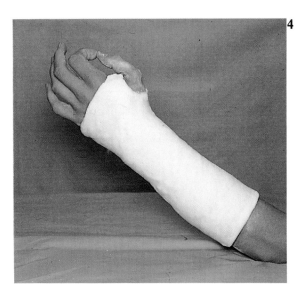

1-4 The forearm is covered in tubular gauze and/or wool bandage (**1**). An assistant may support the fingers and thumb. A 10 cm (4 in) plaster bandage is dipped in water and wrapped smoothly over the padding from knuckles to below the elbow (**2**). The plaster passing between the thumb and index finger is moulded to allow full opposition of the thumb and index finger.

When the wet plaster bandage is about 6 layers thick; the fracture site can be moulded into full reduction (**3**). As the plaster hardens the distal and proximal cuffs of gauze/padding are turned back to form smooth edges. A final layer of plaster bandage can be used to give a uniform surface to the completed cast.

Long arm cast

Fractures of the upper third of both forearm bones are best aligned in supination, fractures of the middle third in mid position and fractures of the lower third in pronation. Smith's or Barton's fractures are immobilised in supination.

Requirements   Tubular gauze; 1 - 2 rolls of 10 cm (4 in) wool bandage; 4 - 5 rolls of 15 cm (6 in) plaster bandage; 1 splint 10 × 30 cm (4 × 12 in) × 5 layers to reinforce elbow.

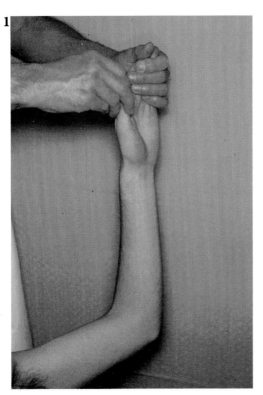

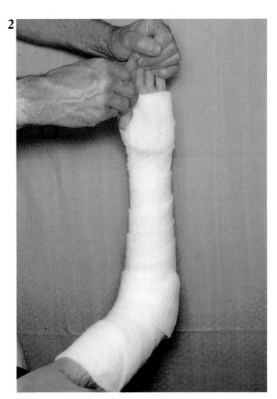

1 & 2   The fracture is usually well aligned if the forearm is held vertically by the assistant gripping the fingers in one hand and the thumb with the other hand. Usually the patient is lying down and anaesthetised. The assistant can control the position of the shoulder and elbow as well as the rotation of the forearm. The arm is encircled by wool bandage to protect the skeletal prominences and to allow for post reduction swelling. The elbow should be held at a right angle.

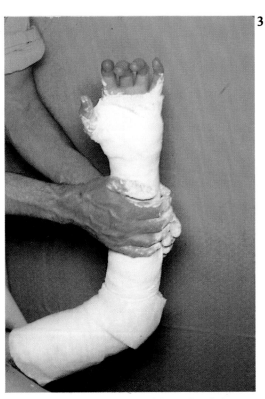

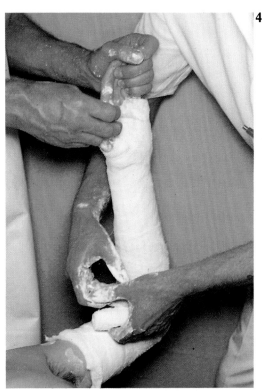

3   The forearm is covered with 2 rolls of plaster bandage and as it sets the manipulator can correct the alignment of the forearm and can impart an oval cross section to the cast.

4   The upper arm is then covered by 2 rolls of plaster bandage. The point of the elbow is often reinforced by a posterior plaster splint and care should be taken not to have too great a thickness of plaster in the front of the elbow. The plaster is finished by turning down the padding at the proximal and distal margins and smoothing the surface.

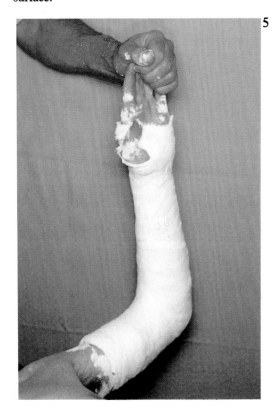

5   The thumb and fingers are allowed complete freedom. The elbow is immobilised at a right angle. (This is partly concealed by the angle of this picture.)

Elbow splint (slab)

Elbow splints (slabs) are used to support injuries around the elbow. The degree of elbow flexion required varies with the nature of the injury. Elbow splints are usually applied posteriorly from shoulder level to wrist or knuckles but there is considerable leverage at the elbow joint so that a supporting splint of plaster is needed across the outer side of the elbow. In comparison to long arm casts they give a margin of safety for the circulation if there is much swelling as they can be loosened quite easily by cutting the surrounding bandage and padding.

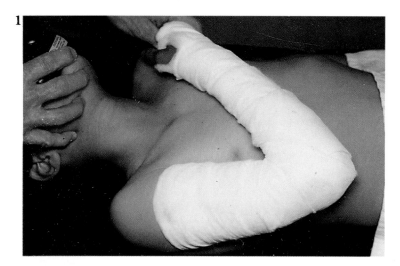

Requirements Tubular gauze; 1 roll of 10 cm (4 in) wool bandage; 1 splint 15 cm (6 in) × 8 layers measuring the length from axilla to knuckles; 1 splint 10 cm (4 in) × 5 layers × 20 cm (8 in); 1 roll 10 cm (4 in) cotton bandage.

1   The arm is padded by the application of wool (or a similar material). Extra padding is required under the point of the elbow. This child's elbow is being held in a position of flexion to immobilise a supra-condylar fracture of the humerus.

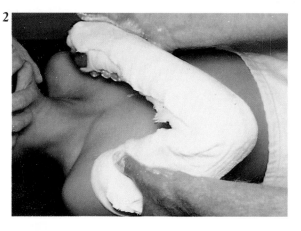

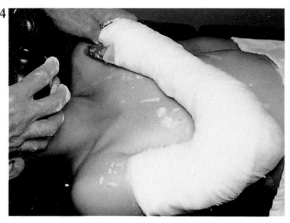

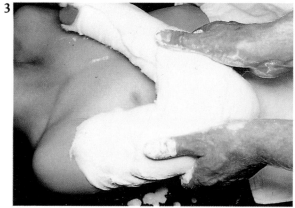

2   The uninjured arm is measured from the axilla to the knuckles and a splint of this length is made from 15 cm (6 in) wide bandage 8 layers thick. An assistant holds the arm in position while the splint is laid on the posterior aspect of the arm from axilla to knuckles.

3   A second shorter splint is made from 10 cm (4 in) bandage about 25 cm (10 in) long and 5 layers thick. This splint is laid across the outer side of the elbow. This reinforces a weak point in the first splint.

4   The splints are held in place with a cotton bandage. It is mandatory to leave a gap in the padding and bandage over the antero-lateral aspect to enable the radial pulse to be felt. The presence of the pulse in most cases confirms that the circulation to the hand is adequate.

Humeral U splint (slab)

Closed fractures of the humeral shaft can be splinted by the application of a plaster splint bent as a U over the lateral and medial surfaces of the upper arm. General anaesthesia is almost never required although analgesia by mouth or injection is useful. Two assistants are required to support the patient's arm and to hold the plaster splint in place.

Requirements Tubular gauze; 1 roll of 10 cm (4 in) wool bandage; 1 splint 15 cm (6 in) × 6 layers measuring twice the length of the upper arm; 1 roll 15 cm (6 in) cotton bandage; 1 collar and cuff sling.

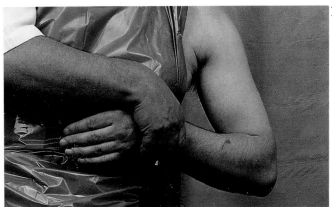

1   The sitting patient should be asked to lean towards the injury so that the fractured arm hangs vertically, thus giving access to the axilla. The plaster splint will pass from the axilla around the elbow to the outer aspect of the shoulder. The length can be measured using a tape and a splint constructed from 15 cm (6 in) wide plaster about 8 - 10 layers thick.

63

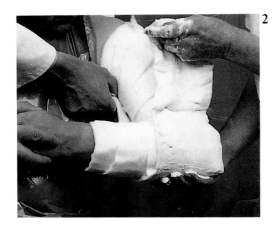

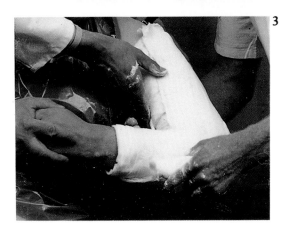

2   The upper arm is wrapped in padding and the plaster splint is applied. The assistant holds the inner part towards the armpit.

3   The U splint is held in position with a cotton bandage.

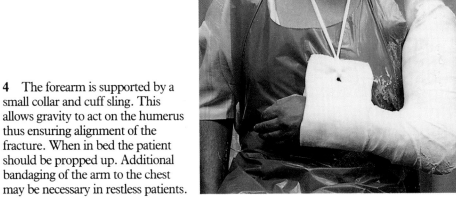

4   The forearm is supported by a small collar and cuff sling. This allows gravity to act on the humerus thus ensuring alignment of the fracture. When in bed the patient should be propped up. Additional bandaging of the arm to the chest may be necessary in restless patients.

Shoulder spica

The cast is applied to patients who have suffered a displaced fracture of the neck of the humerus or who have had an operation around the shoulder joint (i.e. a repair of the rotator cuff or an arthrodesis of the shoulder). It is not often used but is superior to the old-fashioned removable 'aeroplane' splint of wire and leather.

The strut arrangement economises in plaster (and weight) but makes it impossible for the patient to wear a jacket, jersey or shirt unless the sleeve has been removed. The alternative is to support the arm with strong splints of plaster up the side of the trunk moulded in to the armpit and extending along the arm. This adds to the weight of the plaster but makes dressing easier.

Requirements Body stocking and tubular gauze; Adhesive felt; Thin strut of wood; 2 - 4 rolls of 15 cm (6 in) plaster bandage; 3 splints 20 cm (8 in) wide 8 layers thick for trunk; 2 rolls 7.5 cm (3 in) plaster bandage.

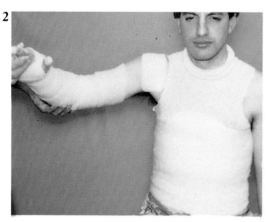

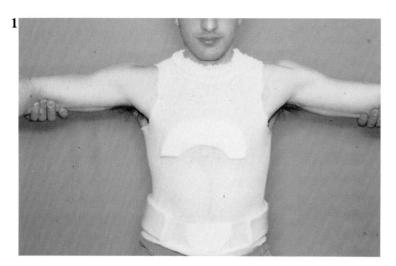

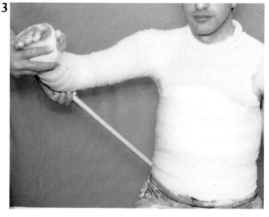

1   The patient is seated on a stool with assistants holding the arms outstretched. A body stocking of tube gauze is applied with pads of adhesive felt to protect the iliac crests, the pubis and the upper sternum

2   A body cast is applied with rolls of plaster bandage [15 or 20 cm (6 or 8 in)] reinforced by 2 or 3 circular splints of 15 or 20 cm (6 or 8 in) width and 8 layers thick (see application of lumbar jacket, page 46). A gauze dressing is applied to any wound or incision on the top of the shoulder. The affected arm is covered in a layer of padding. Particular attention should be directed to padding the elbow and wrist.

3   The chief support of the arm in the outstretched position is a strut of wood approximately 2 cm (¾ in) in diameter. The length is adjusted to fit from waist to elbow. A common position for the shoulder joint and arm is 60° abduction, 60° forward flexion and 60° external rotation.

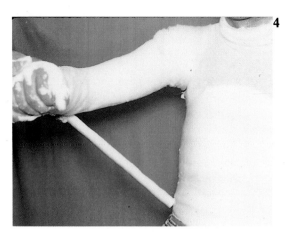

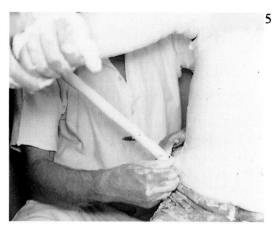

4 The arm and wooden strut are plastered with 15 cm (6 in) rolls of plaster bandage. The wrist is supported in slight dorsiflexion and the forearm in neutral rotation.

5 The strut is anchored in position at the waist and at the elbow with 10 cm (4 in) or 7.5 cm (3 in) plaster bandage. The position of the shoulder is finally adjusted at this time.

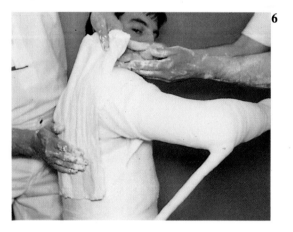

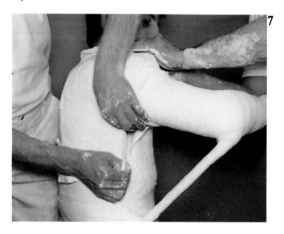

6 Plaster splints and bandages are used to fill the gaps between body cast and arm cast at the shoulder but leaving a ventilation hole at the axilla.

7 The plaster is smoothed to conform to the shape of the shoulder and armpit.

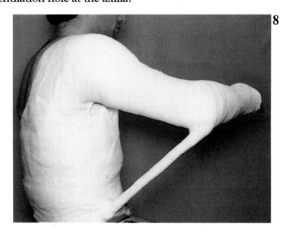

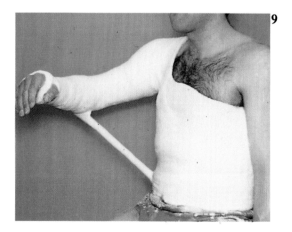

8 The edges of the gauze are turned over the margins of the plaster at the top and bottom of the cast. The whole external surface is smoothed off by encircling rolls of 15 or 20 cm (6 or 8 in) bandage.

9 The final cast should fit comfortably at all points and hold the shoulder firmly in the desired position.

Minerva cast

This type of plaster splint is applied to patients who have had a fracture of, or who have had an operation on, the cervical spine. It is dangerous to use it in those who are quadriplegic, paraplegic or who have insensitive skin beneath the plaster, as large pressure sores can quickly develop.

The patient modelling the plaster has skull tongs in place with traction applied to keep the cervical spine in the required position with minimum difficulty. It is not practical to try to apply this plaster with the patient horizontal as it will not fit properly when the patient becomes vertical. Minerva jackets are not often applied now as they are cumbersome and uncomfortable. The alternative is a halo skull ring attached to a plaster/plastic body jacket or to a pelvic ring.

Requirements Body stocking; Adhesive felt; 2 - 4 rolls of 15 cm (6 in) wool bandage; 4 - 6 rolls of 15 cm (6 in) plaster bandage; 3 splints 20 cm (8 in) wide 8 layers thick for trunk; 2 splints 10 cm (4 in) wide 8 layers thick for shoulders; 1 splint 20 cm (8 in) wide 8 layers thick for neck; 3 splints 5 cm (2 in) wide 8 layers thick for head and face.

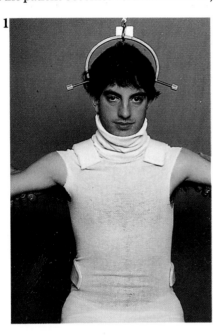

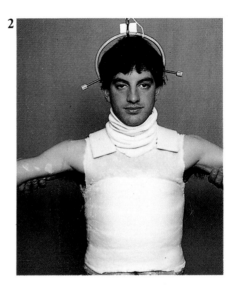

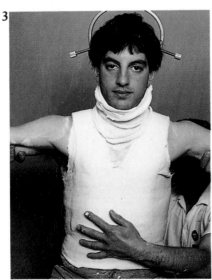

1-3 The patient sits on a stool with skull traction attached to an overhead beam, pulley or ring. This keeps his cervical spine in the neutral position. His arms are supported in the outstretched position by assistants. A body stocking of tube gauze is applied to cover his trunk. A second stocking will cover his neck, face and head at a later stage; this can be left rolled around his neck. Adhesive felt pads are cut and applied to the iliac crests and shoulders where the body cast will press most firmly (**1**). A body cast is applied with rolls of plaster wound around the trunk. An additional 2 or 3 circular splints 6 - 8 layers thick are applied horizontally (**2**). These should be measured to fit the circumference of the trunk. (See application of lumbar jacket, page 46). The distance from the lower ribs is measured from front to back over the shoulders. Two plaster splints 10 cm (4 in) wide and 8 layers thick are then prepared and laid over the shoulders (**3**). Their attachment to the body cast should be carefully smoothed off to eliminate bubbles and to secure a strong union of the parts of the plaster.

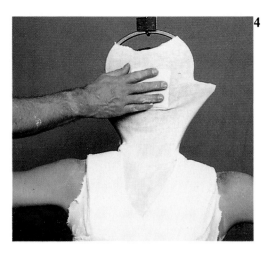

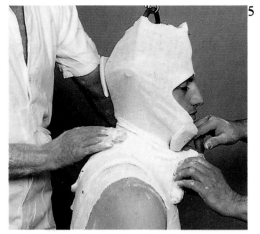

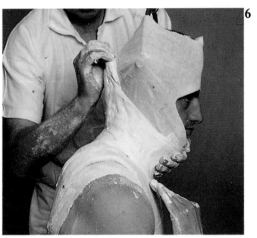

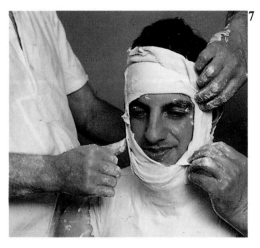

67

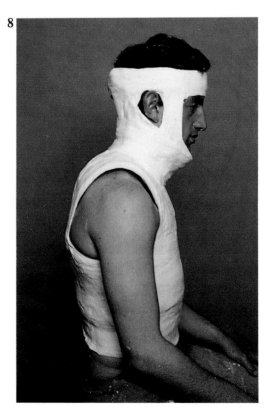

4 & 5 The tube gauze is drawn up over the head and face. A hole is cut for the eyes and nose in front and pads of adhesive felt are fitted over the occiput and under the jaw. Plaster bandages now encircle the neck and are moulded to the chin.

6 & 7 A plaster splint 20 cm (8 in) wide, 8 layers thick and 25 cm (10 in) long is applied vertically from the occiput to between the shoulder blades. This is smoothed into position to fit the shape of the patient's shoulders, neck and head. The head and neck are now supported and the skull tongs removed. The circumference of the head is measured and a plaster splint, 5 cm (2 in) wide and 6 layers thick is prepared, to encircle the head at occiput-forehead level. Two smaller splints, 5 cm (2 in) wide and 6 layers thick, are used vertically in front of the ears.

8 The gauze is trimmed and turned back to produce a smooth edge around the margins of the plaster. Particular attention is paid to the margins around the ears and face. The whole superficial surface of the Minerva cast is smoothed off by encircling turns of plaster bandages 15 or 20 cm (6 or 8 in) wide.

Further reading

History
Cameron D M 1961 Americal Journal of Ortho-
paedics. 3:8

Mechanical properties of plaster bandages
Schmidt V E et al 1973 Biomechanics 6:173
Luck J V 1944 Journal of the American Medical
Association. 124:23

Index